Bedside
PSYCHIATRY

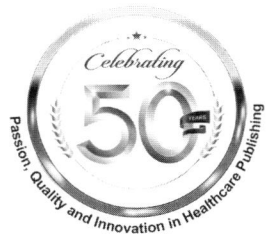

Bedside PSYCHIATRY

Arabinda N Chowdhury
MBBS MD FAMS PhD FAMS FRCPsych PhD (Soc Anthropology) DSc Psychoanalyst
Consultant Psychiatrist
Leicestershire Partnership NHS Trust, UK

Edited by
The Publication Subcommittee
Indian Psychiatric Society

PK Singh (Chairperson)
Shahul Ameen (Co-Chairperson)
Naresh Nebhinani (Convenor)

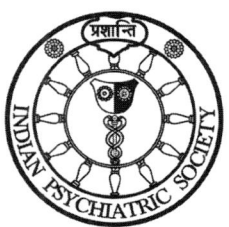

Indian Psychiatric Society Publication

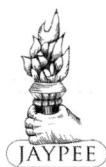

JAYPEE BROTHERS MEDICAL PUBLISHERS
The Health Sciences Publisher
New Delhi | London | Panama

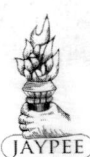 **Jaypee Brothers Medical Publishers (P) Ltd.**

Headquarters
Jaypee Brothers Medical Publishers (P) Ltd
4838/24, Ansari Road, Daryaganj
New Delhi 110 002, India
Phone: +91-11-43574357
Fax: +91-11-43574314
E-mail: jaypee@jaypeebrothers.com

Overseas Offices

JP Medical Ltd
83 Victoria Street, London
SW1H 0HW (UK)
Phone: +44 20 3170 8910
Fax: +44 (0)20 3008 6180
E-mail: info@jpmedpub.com

Jaypee-Highlights Medical Publishers Inc
City of Knowledge, Bld. 235, 2nd Floor
Clayton, Panama City, Panama
Phone: +1 507-301-0496
Fax: +1 507-301-0499
E-mail: cservice@jphmedical.com

Jaypee Brothers Medical Publishers (P) Ltd
Bhotahity, Kathmandu, Nepal
Phone: +977-9741283608
E-mail: kathmandu@jaypeebrothers.com

Website: www.jaypeebrothers.com
Website: www.jaypeedigital.com

© 2019, Jaypee Brothers Medical Publishers and Indian Psychiatric Society

The views and opinions expressed in this book are solely those of the original contributor(s)/author(s) and do not necessarily represent those of editor(s) of the book.

All rights reserved. No part of this publication may be reproduced, stored or transmitted in any form or by any means, electronic, mechanical, photocopying, recording or otherwise, without the prior permission in writing of the publishers.

All brand names and product names used in this book are trade names, service marks, trademarks or registered trademarks of their respective owners. The publisher is not associated with any product or vendor mentioned in this book.

Medical knowledge and practice change constantly. This book is designed to provide accurate, authoritative information about the subject matter in question. However, readers are advised to check the most current information available on procedures included and check information from the manufacturer of each product to be administered, to verify the recommended dose, formula, method and duration of administration, adverse effects and contraindications. It is the responsibility of the practitioner to take all appropriate safety precautions. Neither the publisher nor the author(s)/editor(s) assume any liability for any injury and/or damage to persons or property arising from or related to use of material in this book.

This book is sold on the understanding that the publisher is not engaged in providing professional medical services. If such advice or services are required, the services of a competent medical professional should be sought.

Every effort has been made where necessary to contact holders of copyright to obtain permission to reproduce copyright material. If any have been inadvertently overlooked, the publisher will be pleased to make the necessary arrangements at the first opportunity. The **CD/DVD-ROM** (if any) provided in the sealed envelope with this book is complimentary and free of cost. **Not meant for sale.**

Inquiries for bulk sales may be solicited at: jaypee@jaypeebrothers.com

Bedside Psychiatry

First Edition: **2019**

ISBN: 978-93-5270-985-4

Printed at Rajkamal Electric Press, Kundli, Haryana.

Dedicated to
Our psychiatry trainees

Message

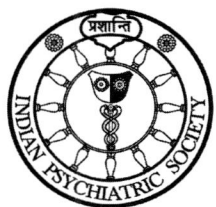

Since its birth Indian Psychiatric Society has remained committed to and proactive in imparting knowledge of psychiatry to the medical undergraduates, postgraduates and working professionals. In recent times, this role has been augmented.

Our CMEs, Conferences and respectably indexed Journal, the Indian Journal of Psychiatry have often made historic contributions. For last few years, our Publication Committee has been actively working on bringing out quality books suitable for Indian subcontinent. Two such books, already published, have been received very well.

The present volume, *Bedside Psychiatry*, has been uniquely designed for all medical graduates who are being trained in Psychiatry. Its approach is practical, covering almost all areas of psychiatric interview and examination. Going through it, one can see that this book is much more than just another a clinical handbook. It contains brief information about all psychiatric disorders. To us it appears as a mini *Textbook of Psychiatry*. The author and Professor Arabinda N Chowdhury, an accomplished academician and clinician, who has worked in India and abroad in important positions. This book embodies not only the available knowledge but also his personal clinical experience. We thank Professor Arabinda N Chowdhury for writing this book for Indian Psychiatric Society. This is the first time that Indian Psychiatric Society has undertaken publication of a book written independently by an author, which is getting published under its auspices. However, it has been editorially reviewed by our Publication Committee.

We congratulate and put on record our sincere thanks to our Publication Committee headed by Professor PK Singh. Professor PK Singh, Drs Shahul Ameen and Naresh Nebhinani have devoted lot of their time in editing this book to enhance its clarity and usefulness.

The Indian Psychiatric Society is grateful to M/s Jaypee Brothers Medical Publishers (P) Ltd, New Delhi, India. for their help and support for quality production. We especially acknowledge the contribution of Ms Chetna Malhotra Vohra (Associate Director—Content Strategy) and Prerna Bajaj (Development Editor).

Ajit V Bhide
President

Mrugesh Vaishnav
President Elect

Vinay Kumar
Hon General Secretary

Foreword

I am honored to provide this foreword. Dr Arabinda N Chowdhury joined the NHS as a Consultant Psychiatrist in 2006. Prior to that, he was Professor and Head, Department of Psychiatry, Institute of Postgraduate Medical Education and Research, and Superintendent of Institute of Psychiatry, Kolkata, West Bengal, India.

Dr Arabinda N Chowdhury has written chapters in books on cultural competency, done several international projects, and is the person who has published the most articles on a culture-bound syndrome 'Koro'. He has extensive experience in running and establishing services in psychiatry.

Despite all his achievements, he is one of the most humble person I have met to date. As part of his passion and self-commitment to create psychiatrists of the highest caliber, he has worked extensively on this book, which is a great resource of knowledge and a pleasure to read. It assimilates information from several aspects. One who reads it will be able to develop both an extensive knowledge and skills base in psychiatry; while also learning the importance of listening and being a caring doctor who is understanding and sensitive to the person who seeks their help. What usually takes psychiatrists years to learn has been summarized proficiently in a book less than 200 pages. This is a treasure for psychiatrists in training and gives the experienced psychiatrists a great way to refresh their knowledge and skills.

In 'Bedside Psychiatry', Dr Arabinda N Chowdhury skillfully draws together the key elements needed to successfully implement the art and science of clinical assessment of a patient. He begins with an introduction to the interview itself with reference to goals, process, and the key components of the physician-patient relationship. *Chapter 2*: History—is a guide to taking a comprehensive and thorough history. *Chapter 3*: Examination—emphasizes the importance of physical, central nervous system, and Mental State Examination (MSE) in a psychiatric evaluation.

The chapter on Mental State Examination, as you would expect, gets particular attention. *Chapter 3* concentrates on the traditional Mental State Examination including clarification and explanation of phenomenology. *Chapter 4* consists of Diagnostic Formulation, Risk Assessments, Mental Capacity Assessment and Treatment Planning, Safeguarding, and Safe Prescribing. Appendices (Appendix 1 to 38) provide additional useful clinical reference material.

I hope Arabinda N you enjoy this book as much as I have and will highly recommend it.

Fabida Noushad
Consultant Psychiatrist in Assertive Outreach Team and Pave Team
Deputy Clinical Director, Adult Mental Health Services
Leicestershire Partnership NHS Trust and
Royal College Regional Advisor for Leicestershire
Northamptonshire and Rutland
OSL House, East Link, Meridian
Leicestershire, LE19 1XU, UK

Preview

Greetings and welcome to all the readers who are glancing through the page of this unique and extraordinary book. This is for the first time that the Publication Committee of Indian Psychiatric Society (IPS) has undertaken the task of publishing a book written independently by one of our own colleagues and a member of the IPS fraternity. This book is being published by the leading medical publication house of the country M/s Jaypee Brothers Medical Publishers (P) Ltd, New Delhi, India. Being a first-time event, there was no precedence. Therefore, a completely new strategy and mechanism had to be evolved to set a trend for the future. It was decided, with the approval of the Executive Council of the IPS, that all such books, which are written independently by various authors on their own but are intended to be published under IPS banner, shall be subjected to an editorial review by a committee set up by the Publication Committee. In the case of Professor Arabinda N Chowdhury's book, for practical reasons, this task was done by the Publication Committee itself.

It is my pleasure to introduce this book, *Bedside Psychiatry*, to a very wide readership, which certainly will receive great acceptance because of its everyday utility. This book is essentially an updated and improvised version of his previously published book, *Psychiatric Interview*. The name change was affected with a view to make it more representative of the broad range of contents included in the book. This book is a distillate of Professor Chowdhury's lifetime experience with psychiatric patients and also the psychiatry trainees to whom the book has justifiably been dedicated. This book certainly has a personal touch of the author in the sense that many aspects of the major headings of mental state examination and management plan have a nonconventional dimension added to it. The process of editorial review by the Publication Committee has not made any significant changes in the finer organization or the actual contents of the book. They have respected the author's jurisdiction over these areas. The Publication Committee has limited itself to the general organization of the book, smoothening of corners at places, enhancing consistency, and ensuring flow of the book.

Bedside Psychiatry brings it much closer to the mainstream disciplines of modern medicine. The inclusion of certain amount of theoretical information as appendix, which is of immediate relevance to the clinician, also adds to the value of the book. *Bedside psychiatry* includes skills of collecting most relevant and valid piece of information from patients and their attendants, further supplementing this information by systematic and insightful physical and mental state assessment, and then making a diagnostic formulation, undertaking required biomedical investigations, and psychometric evaluation leading to a management plan; furthermore, how to implement this plan with due care and expertise.

It has been our pleasure and also privilege to be associated with this task and thereby gain insight and experience in return. We express our most sincere good wishes for wider circulation, acceptance, and readership of this book. We pray that may the publication of this book trigger the arrival of many more even higher quality books from our most talented psychiatric fraternity of Indian Psychiatric Society (IPS).

Long live IPS.

PK Singh
Professor and Head
Department of Psychiatry
Patna Medical College and Hospital
Patna, Bihar, India

Shahul Ameen
Consultant Psychiatrist
St Thomas Hospital
Changanacherry, Kerala, India

Naresh Nebhinani
Associate Professor
Department of Psychiatry
All India Institute of Medical Sciences
Jodhpur, Rajasthan, India

Preface

The psychiatric interview and mental state examination are the key elements of clinical psychiatry. Psychiatric trainees should have an easy-to-use interview and examination format, keeping all the relevant information on mental symptomatology in their mind. This is a brief compilation of all the relevant information usually needed for day-to-day psychiatric evaluation in adult psychiatry. This compilation helps the trainees to get all the important issues relating to examination and treatment planning along with their duties and obligation in a comprehensive manner and helps them to equip with some running clinical oral questions as well. Alongside with the practical clinical examination procedure, the relevant theoretical issues are provided in the 'Appendix' to offer a comprehensive insight about the clinical items.

I am deeply thankful to Dr Fabida Noushad for writing the 'Foreword' for this book. I am expressing my thanks to Dr Rajesh Jacob, Dr John Burke, and Dr M Chawala, all were former consultant psychiatrists of Northamptonshire Healthcare NHS Foundation Trust, for their critical review of the primary draft. I am obligated to my wife Dr Shyamali Chowdhury and daughter Dr Monali Chowdhury for their generous allowance of sufficient academic time during the initial phase of the writing.

I am very thankful to all my past postgraduate students, who over the years, helped me to learn and particularly to Drs KD Sen, Piyal Sen, VG Jhanwar, Amit Bhattacharya, Saikat Basu, S Bhakta, Arabinda Brahma, Sayanti Ghosh, and research coordinator Dr Sohini Banerjee from India. I am also grateful for what I imbibed from my colleagues in the UK, including Dr Anand Madasamy and trainees Shiva Margani, Fabian Motsi, and J Butler. I take the opportunity to express my sincere thanks to three of my colleagues who always supported me in my work: Professor Manoj Bhattacharrya, Former Dean, University College of Medicine, Calcutta University, Kolkata; Professor Makhanlal Saha, Department of Surgery, IPGME and R, Kolkata; and Dr Ajoy Chakraborty, DHS, Government of West Bengal. I must thank Dr Sayanti Ghosh, now Associate Professor of Psychiatry, NRS Medical College in Kolkata, Dr Sohini Banerjee, Assistant Epidemiologist, Care, Bihar, for stringently reviewing of the present draft with suggestions. I am also grateful to Dr Nilanjana Ray, Consultant Pediatrician, London North West University Hospitals NHS Trust, and Dr Samrat Sen Gupta, Consultant Psychiatrist, Broadmoor Hospital, Berkshire, for reviewing the draft and Chandana Chatterjee and Medha Dube for their help in the copy editing of the draft. Lastly, I would like to express my deep gratitude and sincere thanks to the Publication Committee of IPS for their kindness to publish this book. I feel honored by their acceptance, valuable suggestions, and compliments. My special thanks to Professor PK Singh, Chairperson, Publication Committee, for his continued support, constructive suggestion and critical comments on the design and content of the book. I am also thankful to two of our junior colleagues, Drs Shahul Ameen and Dr Naresh Nebhinani who very carefully reviewed the draft with their suggestion.

If this compilation benefits our adult mental health trainees, then this attempt would have been worthwhile.

Arabinda N Chowdhury

Contents

SECTION 1: INTERVIEW, CLINICAL EXAMINATION AND MANAGEMENT

Chapter 1	The Basics	3
Chapter 2	Psychiatric History	14
Chapter 3	Clinical Examination	26
Chapter 4	Additional Evaluation, Management and Related Issues	54

SECTION 2: APPENDICES

Appendix 1	History of Present Complaints	65
Appendix 2	Genogram	66
Appendix 3	Premenstrual Syndrome	67
Appendix 4	Premorbid Personality	68
Appendix 5	Cultural Assessment in Psychiatry	70
Appendix 6	Physical Health Monitoring in Mental Health	74
Appendix 7	Central Nervous System Examination	76
Appendix 8	General Appearance and Behavior	78
Appendix 9	Language Evaluation	80
Appendix 10	Voice and Speech	82
Appendix 11	Catatonia	84
Appendix 12	Mood and Affect	86
Appendix 13	Formal Thought Disorder	91
Appendix 14	Possession of Thought	92
Appendix 15	Non-delusional Thoughts	93
Appendix 16	Delusional Thoughts	98
Appendix 17	Disorders of Perception	104
Appendix 18	Disorder of Identity and Will	117
Appendix 19	Attention and Concentration	120
Appendix 20	Memory	121
Appendix 21	Information and Intelligence	125
Appendix 22	Risk Factors for Violence in Psychosis	126
Appendix 23	Interview of Specific Patients and Situations	128
Appendix 24	Clinical Risk Management	135
Appendix 25	Cognitive State Assessment for Organic Brain Disease and Some Neurological Examinations	138

Appendix 26	Grief, Bereavement and Complicated Grief	**147**
Appendix 27	Diagnostic and Statistical Manual of Mental Disorders (DSM-5)	**149**
Appendix 28	International Classification of Diseases, 10th Revision, WHO (1992)	**151**
Appendix 29	Personality Disorders	**154**
Appendix 30	Ego Defense Mechanisms	**158**
Appendix 31	Some Pioneers of Psychoanalytical Psychiatry	**165**
Appendix 32	Psychiatric Report	**168**
Appendix 33	Commonly Used Rating Scales in Psychiatry	**170**
Appendix 34	Commonly Used Laboratory Tests in Psychiatry	**174**
Appendix 35	Electrocardiogram	**177**
Appendix 36	Some Clinical Syndromes	**181**
Appendix 37	Some Commonly Used Terms/Conditions in Clinical Psychiatry	**183**
Appendix 38	Mental Healthcare Act, 2017 (India)	**189**

Bibliography   **193**
Index   **200**

Section 1

Interview, Clinical Examination and Management

Chapter 1   The Basics
Chapter 2   Psychiatric History
Chapter 3   Clinical Examination
Chapter 4   Additional Evaluation, Management and related issues

Chapter 1

The Basics

■ THE PSYCHIATRIC INTERVIEW

The psychiatric interview is one of the key areas of clinical psychiatry. Developing the skill of interviewing entails continued learning. The nature of every psychiatric interview is unique; and psychiatric residents or medical officers should acquire the skill of interviewing through repeated experience overtime. In the following discussion, the "interviewer" is referred to as psychiatrist.

The psychiatric interview is a creative activity and it is a study of movement and change over the course of time. It is the single most important method of arriving at an understanding of patients who exhibit signs and symptoms of mental disorders. The most distinctive features of the psychiatric interview include examining the individual's feelings about the significant events in his/her life, identifying the significant persons and their relationship with the patient in the course of his/her life, and identifying and tracing the major influences on the biological, social, and psychological development of the individual. It should always be remembered that though the psychiatric interview focuses primarily on a diagnostic formulation, it should help to understand a human being who is in distress. So, the main areas of focus of a psychiatric interview should include the following:
- The patient's psychological makeup
- The patient's perception about his/her environment
- The significant social, religious, and cultural influences on his/her life
- The conscious and unconscious motivations behind the patient's behavior
- The patient's ego, strengths and weakness
- The coping strategies used by the patient
- The patient's defense mechanisms and disposition
- Social support and stressors
- The patient's perception of the current distress and ways of solving it
- The patient's perception of the self and the world.

The psychiatric interview, in addition to eliciting cross-sectional data in relation to the diagnosis and developmental perspective of the patient is also a potentially healing event in which the patient benefits a therapeutic goal by revealing himself or herself in the context of a trusting and nonjudgmental relationship with his/her psychiatrist.

Preparing Yourself for the Interview
- *Listen well:* Listen to what the patient says and show that you are listening.
- *Dress appropriately:* Dressing smartly, tidily, and respectably always matters. Always display your ID badge.
- *Nonjudgmental attitude*: Often, the things uncovered during an interview may conflict with your own constructs of normality or acceptability. Make a conscious effort not to come across as judgmental—whatever the patient says.
- *Flexibility:* Make it clear to the patient from the start that he/she can request a break or end the interview at any time.
- *Friendly and empathetic attitude*: This is one of the key factors for a productive psychiatric interview.
   Some important considerations to be kept in mind before starting the interview are:
- Goal and purpose of the interview
- Interview process
- Physician–patient relationship.

Goal of the Interview
Whatever the purpose of the interview, be it diagnostic, or mental health certification for the judiciary or clinical review, the psychiatrist must accept the patient as a human being and respect his/her value system and integrity as a person. The psychiatrist must be on a "curious mode" and should try to understand the patient's distress profile against the background of his/her sociocultural milieu. It should be remembered that the skill of good psychiatric history taking is an art that must depict a distressed person's life story coherently, obviously with an overall clinical perspective.

The psychiatric interview attempts to seek answers to several basic questions about the patient and his/her presenting problems or distress. The psychiatrist should proceed with a general frame of reference in mind for the interview regarding the following issues:
- Does the patient have a psychiatric disorder or mental health problem?
- How severe is the disorder or the condition?
- What is the probable diagnosis?
- Are there abnormalities in brain function?
- What biological factors contribute to the present problem?
- What psychological factors contribute to the present problem?
- What environmental factors contribute to the present problem?
- What is the patient's baseline level of functioning?
- What is the patient's motivation and capacity in terms of treatment?
- What management plans that suit this patient best?
- Does the patient's current behavior posing any risk to self or to others and how best the risk can be managed?

Interview Process

Factors that affect the Interview: A number of factors can influence the interview process and thus influence the alliance and yield of the relevant information. The interviewer must take into account the following factors that may affect the interview:
- The extent of the patient's physical or emotional distress
- The patient's cognitive capacities
- The emotionally based biases of the patients (transference)
- The emotionally based biases of the interviewer (countertransference)
- Situational factors
- Racial, ethnic, and cultural factors or background.

General Features of the Psychiatric Interview:
- Setting
- Verbal communication
- Nonverbal communication
- Listening and observation
- Attitude and behavior of the interviewer.

Listening skill (Mohl, 2004): Patients are storytellers who have the hope of being heard and properly understood. The listeners are the physicians who are expected to listen actively and develop a new level of understanding of their patients. Listening enhances all other skills in diagnosis—the therapeutic alliance and communication. So, listening becomes one of the central skills in clinical psychiatry. Psychiatrists, more than any other physicians, must constantly listen in diverse ways: symptomatically, narratively and experientially, behaviorally, interpersonally, cognitively, cross-culturally, and from a systems perspective.

Three factors are important in quantifying the listening:
1. Listening is more than just listening—the psychiatrist must be acquainted with the patient's cultural biogrammar, so that he/she can understand the language, symbolic meaning of the symptoms, family background, and forces of the social system.
2. The psychiatrist must have an immediate grasp of all sorts of symptoms and syndromes readily available in mind.
3. The psychiatrist should hear the patient's story in a variety of flexible ways, so that he/she can correctly pinpoint the symptom(s) and their experience from the narrative.

Many factors influence the ability to listen. The common causes of *blocks* (Mohl, 2004) to effective listening are as follows:
- *Patient–psychiatrist's dissimilarity:* Race, sex, culture, religion, regional dialect, and socioeconomic differences.
- *Superficial similarities*: May lead to faulty assumptions of shared meanings.
- *Countertransference*: Psychiatrists fail to hear specific content, reminiscent of his/her unresolved conflicts.
- *External forces*: Treatment set-up, scarcity of time, limited space, or privacy and work pressure.
- *Attitudes*: Psychiatrist's cultural value system and his/her emotional state during the interview.

All psychiatrists, regardless of their theoretical position, must develop the skill of listening—the psychodynamic psychiatrists look out for unconscious conflicts; the cognitive psychiatrists look out for the patient's hidden distortions, false beliefs, and assumptions about their environment; behaviorist looks out for hidden associations and maladaptive behavior patterns; and interpersonal psychiatrists look out for stereotypical role definitions, interpersonal conflicts, and deficits in adaptive defenses. Psychiatry is a discipline in which the experience of listening over and over again allows the listener to grow in his/her capacity to hear. *This is one of the qualities of a good psychiatrist.*

Structure of the interview: The interview is a process of detailed inquiry. Its structure depends on its purpose. The day-to-day clinical interview is usually short, open-ended or structured. In some specific situations (for a judicial report or for diagnostic report), we also use highly structured interview formats, which enable us to collect the necessary clinical information to facilitate planning with a reasonable period of time.

Phases of the interview: There may be a single or multiple interviews. Each session has three components: Opening, middle, and closing parts. Opening phase may include an introduction and the collection of the patient's chief complaints and his/her demographic features. Middle phase consists of assessing the major issues of clinical importance. Closing phase consists of treatment planning and a discussion, risk assessment and the patient is given appropriate advice.

Dimensions of Interviewing

The four important issues (Silberman and Certa, 2004) involved here are:
1. *Directiveness*: Directiveness is the natural flow and spontaneity of the interview. Directiveness ensures that the necessary access to information is covered with adequate relevance. The directiveness may be *low, medium,* or *high* and the psychiatrist should intervene accordingly to obtain the desired clinical information. For example, in the case of low directiveness, the nature of the intervention may be repetition, clarification, or open-ended questions. The intervention in the case of moderate directiveness may be the use of examples, interpretation or broad-focus questions. In high directiveness, redirection, changes of topics, and the limit setting are the usual interventions.
2. *Supporting*: Patients differ considerably in the degree of emotional as well as cognitive support they need during the interview. The usual *supportive interventions* are:
    - Encouragement, approval, and reassurance
    - Acknowledgement of affect
    - Empathic statements
    - Nonverbal communication
    - Temporary avoidance of affect–laden topics

    Obstructive interventions are those that impede the flow of information and diminish rapport. They are:
    - Asking biased or judgmental questions and making judgmental statements
    - Asking too many questions and ignoring the patient's lead

- Asking vague questions
- Giving premature advice or reassurance
- Behaving or communicating in a nonverbal manner that shows a lack of interest in the patient.

3. *Fact-feeling orientation*: Interviewers differ in the degree to which they focus on *factual-objective* oriented versus *feeling-and-meaning* oriented information. The psychiatrist should maintain an adequate balance between these three components while taking the patient's history. Fact-oriented interventions are: Asking questions about the symptoms, behavior, and intent, and eliciting medical data. Feeling-oriented interventions are: Asking questions about the patient's feelings in specific situations or comments about emotional issues or patterns and asking questions related to the personal meaning of an event.

4. *Feedback*: Interviewers differ regarding how much of the information gleaned through the interview, impressions obtained or the recommendation they have in mind should be discussed with the patient. The following are a few issues related to feedback to the patient:
   - Sharing subjective reactions
   - Imparting scientific information
   - Proposing a formulation
   - Discussing the treatment plan with information on the side effects of the medication
   - Giving suitable advice regarding risk management
   - Responding to questions.

It is a good medical practice to discuss the salient findings and explain the diagnosis in a simple manner (nonmedical way). Remember not all patients are similar. Some may insist on a particular diagnosis for their own agenda and may be challenging, while some may be satisfied and agree with your explanation. It is your skill and clinical intelligence that may help to resolve the issue. In the event of controversy, consult a senior colleague for a second opinion.

Physician–Patient Relationship

Building a cooperative and trusting relationship with patients is a key factor in enabling psychiatrists to foster the healing process. A psychiatrist should have the ability to sustain a professional attitude and to practice within a set of ethical boundaries. The psychiatrist must be well acquainted with the six key principles (Epstein, 1994) of medical ethics:

1. *Beneficence:* Applying one's ability solely for the patient's well-being
2. *Nonmalfeasance*: Avoiding harm to the patient
3. *Autonomy:* Respecting the patient's independence and rights
4. *Justice*: Avoiding prejudicial bias based on the idiosyncrasies of the patient's background, behavior, or life situation
5. *Confidentiality:* Respect for the patient's privacy
6. *Veracity*: Truthfulness with oneself and one's patients.

Boundary Violations: Mental health treatment approaches involve psychiatrists and patients entering into each other's space which means crossing boundaries. Gutheil and Gabbard

(1993) defined boundary violations as the crossing of boundaries that causes injury to the patient. Due to dealing with the patient's emotional turmoil, the psychiatrist becomes an object of projected dependency for the patient. So, from the initial psychiatric interview up to the completion of the treatment regime, the psychiatrist has to maintain a high standard of professional ethics and boundaries in this clinical relationship. The aim of being a good therapeutic friend, without committing any nonsexual or sexual boundary violations, is an issue that the psychiatrist must pay careful attention to and this matter should be of the utmost concern to him/her. The following issues of potential boundary violations should be carefully avoided in psychiatric clinical practice:

- It is undesirable if the treatment plan is not judicious according to the need of the patient, and does not reflect the psychiatrist's wisdom and honest endeavor to follow the *evidence-based clinical approach.*
- Psychiatrists should not relate to the patient as their personal friend.
- Psychiatrists should not accept any gifts or personal favor from their patients.
- Psychiatrists should not maintain any contact with the patient outside the therapy setting.
- Psychiatrists should not try to impress their patient with their personal information.
- Psychiatrists should not have sexual relations or a sexual preoccupation with the patient.

To achieve an optimum therapeutic alliance is the aim of all psychiatric interviews. However, this aim may be hindered by some special problems related to the type of patient. The interviewer should have an insight into the potential problems that can arise during interviews with delusional patients, hostile patients, violent and agitated patients, depressed patients, highly seductive patients, and deceitful patients. Special interviewing skills are required for each situation described above (*Please see Appendix 23, page-128*). There should be adequate resources; arrangements for physical restraint, and seclusion or maintaining a distance. The interviewer must be immune to provocative abuse or infective emotion of grandiosity or the existential despair manifested by depressed patients. The interviewer must remain alert while interviewing seductive patients and should be aware of the legal perspectives while interviewing a deceitful patient. Psychiatric ethics are based on the traditional medical values of trust and commitment to a healing relationship. Recent advances in medical technology and therapeutic dimensions have changed this paradigm of relatedness. Thus, psychiatric and medical ethics are also undergoing changes, but there is no change in the basic theme: "I will never use my medical wisdom to injure or wrong them".

Transference and Countertransference: Transference is the unreasonable displacement of attitudes and feelings (originating in childhood) to other people. This phenomenon is likely to affect the doctor–patient relationship. The patient may unconsciously regard the physician as a parent or a sibling, casting him/her in a caring or antagonistic role. The usual roles are of a nurturing or demanding mother, a protective or punitive father, and a rival sibling. Sometimes, older patients relate to the physician as though they themselves are parents, reversing the roles.

It is important to recognize transference during the interview process. When the patient is exceptionally deferential, hanging onto the interviewer's opinions, singing his/her praises to others, or is easily slighted by a brief or delayed appointment, the interviewer may suspect a *positive* transference. When the patient is unexpectedly hostile, suspicious, or competitive, and there is no reasonable explanation for such antagonism, a *negative* transference is likely. A note of serious caution: A positive transference can become eroticized with the patient falling in love with an idealized parental figure. If the interviewer recognizes this and responds in a professional manner, the patient will go no further. Occasionally, however, the patient may make unscheduled visits, write notes, make telephone calls, or dress seductively which indicates that the matter is more serious. The interviewer should not respond impulsively and should consult a colleague about how to resolve these issues.

Countertransference occurs when a physician irrationally transfers his/her attitudes and feelings (derived from childhood experiences) to a patient. Psychiatric interviewers must be alert about countertransference. They should suspect it whenever they have powerful feelings of affection, protectiveness, fear, frustration, irritation, or hatred, or erotic feelings toward a patient; when they very much look forward to the next appointment; or when they cannot tolerate a particular patient. If the interviewer recognizes these feelings, he/she will be much less likely to respond impulsively with rejection, flight, or self-indulgence. It is always a good practice to seek the help of other colleagues regarding how to proceed in the patient's best interests.

Psychiatrists, psychotherapists, and all other health professionals should be sufficiently aware of boundary violations in their therapeutic engagement with patients and must avoid the following boundary violations (Denman, 2010):
- Showing intimacy, engaging in sex and self-disclosure
- Displaying anger, abusing, or assaulting the patient
- Abusing the patient for dependency needs
- Engaging in financial impropriety and receiving gifts
- Breaching the confidentiality of the case.

Please remember:
- *Treat your patient with the dignity and respect due to a human being*
- *Be polite and gentle in your interactions. Do not be rough and confrontational*
- *Be nonjudgmental in your attitude and approach*
- *Be interested in the patient and his/her concerns*
- *Medicine is an art of healing. History taking is the art, and your wisdom regarding management is the healing. Combine the two skillfully*
- *In the case of any confusion, consult your superior or another psychiatrist*
- *Write everything clearly and legibly. Having good handwriting is a positive quality, not discreditable. All clinical notes should be signed and dated*
- *Always try to follow the prescribed interview format*
- *Each patient is a new challenge adding to your learning*
- *You are the "instrument" for measuring the distress of another human being. Keep the instrument healthy and in sound order; make it reflexive and responsive, so that the quality is always assured and beyond question.*

Your professional identity is dependent on your knowledge, honesty, integrity, concern, and respect for your patients. Always remember that your patients are your strength and resource, as they will help you to be an experienced and skilled expert. This, in turn, brings you recognition and respect in the profession and community at large.

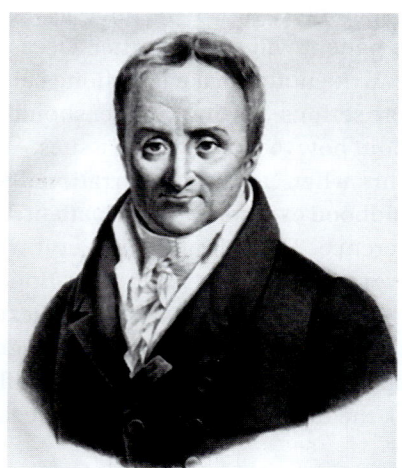

Philippe Pinel (20.04.1745–25.10.1826), a French physician, pioneered the development of a rational and humane psychological approach to the custody and care of mental patients.

■ SOME ETHICAL CONCEPTS OF BINDING VALUES IN CLINICAL CARE

Before taking any clinical responsibility by examining a patient and formulating a diagnosis and treatment, care plan, and risk management, the physician should be aware of and maintains his/her professional/ethical and legal responsibilities toward his/her clients. Very briefly, these are discussed here.

Duty of Care

As a health professional, you have a legal and moral responsibility to keep your clients safe from harm while they are using your service. This responsibility is known as "duty of care". In tort law, a person who violates the duty of care by acting negligently or deliberately is liable for any harm another person suffers as a result of the first person's failure to be reasonably careful.

In a *medical malpractice* case, a doctor's actions are compared to the actions that a reasonable doctor in his field and in the same clinical situation would have taken. Failing to live up to the duty of care is known as a *breach of duty*.

Pandit and Pandit (2009) very clearly stated that what the ambit of Duty of Care is saying. "It is expected that a doctor should carry out necessary investigation or seek a report from the patient. Furthermore, unless it is an emergency, he obtains the informed consent of the patient before proceeding with any major treatment, surgical operation, or even invasive investigation. Failure of a doctor and hospital to discharge this obligation is essentially a tortious liability. A tort is a civil wrong (*right in rem*) as against a contractual obligation (*right in personam*)—a breach that attracts judicial intervention by way of awarding damages. Thus, a patient's right to receive medical attention from doctors and hospitals is essentially a civil right. The relationship takes the shape of a contract to some extent because of informed consent, payment of fee, and performance of surgery/providing treatment, etc. while retaining essential elements of tort".

The duty of care to a patient starts from the moment he/she is accepted for treatment and begins to receive services. Health professionals have a duty of care to their patients, and requires all that is reasonable must be done to secure the best outcome possible. Similarly, health organizations (care providers) have the responsibility to their clients of safeguarding them from any harm or injury they may experience from the service.

Duty of care covers several aspects, such as:
- *Legal*: What does the law suggest we do?
- *Professional/ethical*: What do other workers expect us to do?
- *Organizational*: What does our organization say we should do?
- *Community*: What do the parents/relatives of our patients and other community members expect us to do?
- *Personal*: What do our own beliefs and values suggest we do.

Accountability

"Accountability" is about taking responsibility for one's actions, always ensuring that one is competent to perform the activity that one has been asked to perform, and always putting the patients' interests first. Accountability also means complying with the code of conduct for healthcare workers as per the rules of the health organization or of the land (http://rcnhca.org.uk/46-2/accountability-and-delegation/accountability/).

In practice, this means that whatever one does as a health professional, one should be able to justify it as a sensible course of action. This means that whenever one performs any action:
- One should know why one is doing it
- One should have been properly trained and assessed as being competent to do it
- One should be doing it as part of an agreed plan of care for the patient.

Consent

All clinical contacts should proceed after obtaining the prior consent of the patient. These include the interview, diagnosis, treatment, investigation, organ transplant, research, disclosure of medical records to other professionals, and for teaching and medicolegal purposes. Consent may be given verbally or in writing.

The different types of consent are (Pandit and Pandit, 2009):
- *Express consent*: This may be oral or in writing. Written consent can be considered as superior because of its evidential value.
- *Implied consent*: Consent may be implied by the patient's conduct/body language.
- *Tacit consent*: This means implied consent that is understood without being stated.

- *Surrogate consent*: This consent is given by family members. Generally, courts have held that the consent of family members with the written approval of two physicians protects a patient's interest sufficiently.
- *Advance consent*: This is the consent given by a patient in advance.
- *Proxy consent*: This indicates consent given by an authorized person.
- *Informed consent*: This consent is obtained after explaining all the possible risks, benefits, and side effects of the treatment/medications/surgical procedures to the patient. It is superior to all other forms of consent.

NHS (http://www.nhs.uk/conditions/consent-to-treatment/pages/introduction.aspx) has provided the following guidelines for consent:

For consent to be valid, it must be voluntary and informed, and the person consenting must have the *capacity* to make the decision.

- *Voluntary*: The decision to either consent or not to consent to treatment must be made by the person himself or herself, and must not be influenced by pressure from medical staff, friends, or family.
- *Informed*: The person must be given all the information in terms of what the treatment involves including the benefits and risks, whether there are reasonable alternative treatments and what will happen if treatment does not go ahead.
- *Capacity*: The person must be capable of giving consent which means they understand the information given to them and can use it to make an informed decision.

Confidentiality

Confidentiality is a cornerstone of the clinical encounter. It means not telling anyone, other than those who should or need to know, what a patient has said to the health professional or the problem that they have. It is also important not to show anyone (other than those who should or need to know) an individual's personal notes or computer records. Confidentiality is important because it helps to build trust between the patient and the physician. This trust encourages the patient to disclose their health-related problems to the physician.

The five rules of confidentiality are:
1. Information about patients should be treated confidentially and respectfully.
2. Health professionals should share confidential information when it is needed for the safe and effective care of an individual.
3. Information that is shared for the benefit of the community should be anonymized.
4. An individual's right to object to the sharing of confidential information about them should be respected.
5. Health organizations should put policies, procedures, and systems in place to ensure that confidentiality rules are followed.

(Details of Confidentiality issues may be available in The Data Protection Act (DPA) 1998 at https://www.health-ni.gov.uk/articles/data-protection-act-dpa-1998 and in GMC's document on Laws on disclosure for health and social care purposes at http://www.gmc-uk.org/ guidance/ethical guidance /30639.asp).

STEPS IN CLINICAL PSYCHIATRIC EVALUATION AND INTERVENTION

The following steps are involved in clinical psychiatric evaluation and intervention:
1. *Psychiatric history*:
    - Identification
    - Chief complaint
    - History of present complaints
    - Past psychiatric and medical history
    - Family history
    - Personal history (childhood, adulthood)
    - Premorbid personality
    - Cultural history and assessment
2. *Clinical examinations*:
    - Physical examination
    - Neurological examination
    - Mental state examination
    - Additional clinical issues (risk assessment, capacity assessment).
3. *Investigations* indicated (psychological, neurological, radiological, or laboratory tests)
4. *Extended interview* intended (with family members or other agencies)
5. *Diagnostic formulation with differential diagnosis*
6. *Treatment/care plan including risk management/referral*
7. *Summary findings and follow-up monitoring.*

(However, description in the ensuing pages will follow as per the sequence given in the content page).

Chapter 2

Psychiatric History

■ BEFORE STARTING THE INTERVIEW

- *Be sure about the logistics of the interview setting: Appropriate seating arrangement, privacy, safety, and undisturbed environment.*
- *Greet the patient verbally; introduce yourself and any other people, if present.*
- *Explain the purpose of the interview.*
- *Explain the focus of this interview (e.g. current problems or response to treatments, etc.)*
- *Explain the need to take notes and seek the patient's consent.*
- *If you need to speak to an informant, take the patient's permission.*
- *Sensitive topics such as suicide, sexuality, abuse or forensic history should be asked tactfully and with great skill.*
- *Reassure the patient about confidentiality. The patient should be informed about who will have access to the notes and who will be sent letters relating to this assessment.*
- *Psychiatry/mental health is known to be associated with an age-old stigma—from both social and professional concerns. Many have voiced that the term "patient" is often derogatory and hence it is a good practice to use the term "service user" instead of "patient".*

Be sure about the quality of a good history: The history should be:
- Systematic and coherent with appropriate headings
- Comprehensive with positive features and relevant negative findings
- Reflect the clinical relevance and priorities
- Unnecessary details should be avoided
- Multidimensional in approach, taking consideration of relevant psychological, social, and cultural/spiritual aspects.

Chapter 2: Psychiatric History

■ IDENTIFYING DATA

Clinic registration number:_____ Date:_____
Name:_____ Sex:_____
Date of birth:_____ Age:_____ Ethnicity:_____
Marital status:_____
Education: _____
Occupation: _____
Socioeconomic status: _____
Family (nuclear/extended): _____
Religion: _____
Mother tongue: _____
Address:_____ House number:_____ Street:_____
Country:_____ Post code:_____ Phone number:_____
Nearest relative/caregivers*:_____
Name: _____ Relation:_____
Address and Phone number:
_____
_____

Accompanied by:_____
Purpose of consultation:_____
Referral:_____
History taken by: Name/designation and signature with date:
_____
_____

Note: *"Caregiver" means a person who resides with a person with mental illness and is responsible for providing care to that person and includes a relative or any other person who performs this function either free or with remuneration.

■ CHIEF COMPLAINTS

Chief or presenting complaint: Description of main *current* problem or distress (usually since last 4 weeks) for which the patient is visiting this clinic. The usual question to be asked: "What are the major problems that have been troubling you currently?" or "What are the difficulties that have brought you here?"

Usually, we record the account from the patient, but some situations need corroboration from the accompanying relative or informant. In grossly psychotic patients, the informant may be the only source for getting proper complaints and history. Some of the symptoms relating to beliefs and behavior also need to be cross-checked with family members. It is customary to record the patient's words verbatim without paraphrasing or interpreting them. The account should be recorded in simple and nontechnical language.

- *From patient*: Verbatim—in chronological order with severity and duration of each complaint
- *From informant (collateral information)*: Relevant details in support of the patient's complaints or any valuable additional information in relation to the current distress.

HISTORY OF PRESENT COMPLAINTS

It is the coherent and relevant background history of the development of presenting symptoms. It has two basic components, both of which help as the pointer to the diagnosis:
1. *Symptomatic context:* The way in which the lead symptom points toward the identifiable mental disorder; and
2. *Temporal context*: Nature, extent, and time course of the symptomatology.

Points to be covered:
- Precipitating factors (if any)
- *Mode of onset*: Acute/gradual/not known
- Total duration of illness (in months or weeks)
- *Course of the present complaints*: Continuous/episodic/in remission/exacerbation?/not known
- *History of present complaints*: A narrative account of lead symptom(s), sequence of distress; the impact of symptoms; evaluation of associated symptoms; nature and details of dysfunction
- *Concomitant changes in biological needs/functions*:
  - *Appetite*: No change/mildly or moderately reduced/markedly reduced/enhanced
  - *Libido*: No change/mildly or moderately reduced/markedly reduced/enhanced
  - *Sleep*: Normal/disturbed
- *Treatment history, if any, for the present complaints*: Details with medications used their clinical response/adverse reactions, if any.
- Allergy/drug reaction history.

Note: Please see Appendix 1: page-65.

HISTORY OF PAST ILLNESS

- Past medical illness: Absent/present
- Past surgical illness/operation/accidents: Absent/present
- Past psychiatric illness: Absent/present
- Previous or current medications and *allergies* or side effects, if any
- Record the details—nature, duration, treatment, and outcome of the illness
- A quick medical system probing may be useful to elicit any dysfunction or existing illness: Ask the patient—*have you ever had any problem/difficulties like*:

Body system	Findings
• Headaches, blackouts, or fits?	
• Problems with your vision, hearing, taste?	
• Thyroid problems?	
• Infections or injury?	
• Problems with your breathing or your heart or hypertension?	
• Trouble with urination or passing stools?	
• Joint pain or skin conditions?	
• Difficulties with balance or walking?	

FAMILY HISTORY

A detailed family history is of great importance as family relationships, upbringing, and dynamics can be closely linked to the etiology, management, and prognosis of some mental disorders. In general, the family history aims to establish the following issues:
- To ascertain the *inherited risk* of a psychiatric or medical disorder (note any genetic disorder present in the family)
- To understand the family structure, working and relationships, and any pathology
- To complement the social and personal history.
  Following points to be recorded:
1. Consanguinity in parents: Absent/present
2. Step parents: Yes/No
3. Adopted: Yes/No
4. Parents:

	Father	Mother
Living/present age		
Deceased/at age		
Patient's age at parent's death		
Cause of death		
Education		
Occupation		
Personality		
Relation with patient: poor/bad/usual/good		
History of mental illness*		
History of physical illness*		
History of substance use*		

Note: *Record the detailed account of specific symptoms/diagnosis, course, treatment, and outcome.

5. Siblings: History of any psychiatric illness
6. Family history of suicide
7. Family cohesion and quality of relationship with the patient: Good/bad/usual
8. Family stress: Major illness or accident/bereavement/suicide/separation or divorce
9. Any other relevant information
10. Put the relevant information in a simplified genogram *(Please see Appendix: 2; page-66)*.

PERSONAL HISTORY

1. *Prenatal history*: Nature of mother's pregnancy [planned or unplanned; health status during pregnancy; immunization, history of trauma; drug ingestion (prescribed or abused; use of abortifacient) and any other significant finding].
2. *Birth history*: Normal/abnormal

Order	Only child	First child	Middle child	Last child
Term	Before	Full	After	
Place of delivery	Home	Institution	Other	
Type of delivery	Normal	Forceps	Cesarean	Other
Labor	Normal	Distressed	Prolonged	Other
Cry	Normal	Abnormal: Specify		
Cyanosis/jaundice	Absent	Present: Specify		
Immediate breastfeeding	Yes	No: Reason		
Any other relevant information				

3. *Early childhood (through age 3 years)*:
   - *Feeding habits:* Breastfeed/bottle-fed/age of weaning/eating problems (food fad/pica/others)
   - *Early developments:* Walking/talking/teething/language development/motor development/sleep pattern/object constancy/stranger anxiety/maternal deprivation/separation anxiety
   - *Toilet training:* Age/attitudes of parents/feelings about it/other
   - *Behavioral problems*: Thumb sucking/bedwetting and soiling/temper tantrums/tics/head bumping/rocking/night terrors/fears/nail biting/stammering/truancy/other
   - *Childhood disorders:* Febrile convulsions/seizures/other illness
   - *Temperament as a child*: Shy/restless/overactive/withdrawn/outgoing/timid/athletic/friendly/patterns of play
   - *Milestones of development:* Normal/delayed
4. *Middle childhood (3–11 years)*:
   - *Early school history:* Feeling about going to school/school phobia/adjustment to school
   - *Gender identification:* Normal/abnormal: Specify_____
   - *Peer relations*: Normal/abnormal: Specify_____
   - *Behavioral problems:* (Phobias/bedwetting/fire setting/cruelty to animal/attention or concentration/hyperactivity problem)
5. *Late childhood (puberty through adolescence)*:
   - *Social relationship:* Attitudes toward siblings and schoolmates/number and closeness to friends/leader or follower/participation in group or gang activity/idealized figures/pattern of aggression/other
   - *School history:* Level reached/adjustment with teachers and classmates/favorite study or interest/particular assets or abilities/extracurricular activities/sports/hobbies/scholastic performance—poor, average, good/relation of problems or symptoms to any school period/other like suspension from school for any behavioral problem, etc.

- *Cognitive and motor development*: Learning/reading/intellectual skills/motor skills/other
- *Adolescent emotional or physical problems*: Nightmares/phobias/bedwetting/running away/smoking/alcohol/substance use/delinquency/eating disorders/weight problems/feelings of inferiority or concern for physical look
- *Adolescent turmoil*: Any significant event

6. *Psychosexual history (childhood through adolescence)*:
   - Early curiosity/infantile masturbation/sex play
   - Acquisition of sexual knowledge
   - Attitude of parents toward sex
   - Sexual or physical abuse (detailed history—perpetrator, nature, outcome, safeguarding, etc.)
   - *Onset of puberty:* Feelings about it/kind of preparation/feelings about masturbation/feelings about menarche/development of secondary sexual characters
   - Adolescent sexual activity
   - *Attitude toward opposite sex*: Timid/shy/aggressive/seductive/anxiety
   - *Sexual practices:* Sexual problems/heterosexual or homosexual experiences/paraphilias/promiscuity/orientation preferences

7. *Home situations in childhood and adolescence*: Congenial/broken home/disturbing/others

8. *Any parental lack before 18 years of age*: Dead/separated/habitually absent for more than a year

9. *Adulthood*:
   - *Occupational history:* Applicable/Not applicable
     (Started working at the age of __/Any change of job and reason/Present job—nature and duration __; Satisfaction/work position—rising, falling, static/Work record—good, satisfactory, unsatisfactory/ambition and conflicts/relation with peers and colleagues)
   - *Social history:* Has friends/withdrawn/socializing well. Social mixing/Participation—poor/usual/good. Relationship with people of same and opposite sex/Others___
     Present living conditions/Social support system/Quality of life
   - *Adult sexuality*: Problematic/no problem (*very sensitive part of history taking*)
     Sexual symptoms: Lack of desire/erectile dysfunctions/premature ejaculation/anorgasmia/dyspareunia/vaginismus/impotence/others: present prior to present illness?
     Contracted STD or tested for HIV: Yes/No (details)
     Current sexual preference (orientation): Same sex/opposite sex/both sex
     Sexual practices:
     Coital problems (if any)_____
     Pre- and extramarital sexual relations: Yes/No
     Any conflict or stress related to pregnancy/abortion/infertility
   - *Marital history:*
     Married or living together

Age at marriage___
Consanguineous: No/yes—relation_____
Spouse: Age at marriage, present age, occupation, physical/mental illness?
Marital adjustment: Good/satisfactory/unsatisfactory—specify____
Sexual adjustment: Good/satisfactory/unsatisfactory—specify_____
Family planning/contraceptive measures?
In-laws problems: No/yes
Marital conflict: No/yes
Domestic violence: No/yes—specify
Number of Issues:
History of divorce or separation?

- *Menstrual history:*
Menarche age_____
Periods: Regular or irregular/duration/amount—normal, scanty, excess, spots/premenstrual symptoms/relation of menstruation with present problems/enquire about premenstrual syndrome *(Please see Appendix 3: page-67)*
Amenorrhea (primary/secondary)—present or absent
Menopause: Applicable/not applicable; postmenopausal symptoms?

- *Quick checkbox for personal history*:

1. Birth/infancy	Any positive findings	2. Childhood	Any positive findings
Birth timing and complications		Family relationships in the upbringing	
Breastfed or bottle-fed		Nursery and early schooling	
Any separation from mother		Socializing and befriending	
Growth and developmental targets		Academic and sporting abilities	
Any significant pathology		Any physical/sexual abuse	
3. Adolescence		**4. Adulthood**	
School life and academic achievements		Marital and sexual history (list of past relationships, children, bereavements)	
Pubertal development (physically and psychological)		Occupational history (list of jobs, promotions, satisfaction)	
Peer relationships (including sexual)		Family and support network	
Experimentation with alcohol or drugs, any antisocial behavior		Present financial condition	
Any significant event with potential impact		Future goals and plans	

10. *Self-harm history*: Not applicable/applicable

Number of attempts/date	Method (cutting or burning skin/punching or hitting themselves/poisoning/misuse of drugs or alcohol/deliberate starving (AN) or binge eating)	Outcome

Acute suicidal ideation ever (detail):

Record detailed account of each attempt: An account of circumstances, stress factor present, precautions taken against discovery, preparatory acts (procuring means, warning statements, suicidal note), type and lethality of the method, communication after attempt, the reason for the attempt and outcome (hospitalization and stay).

11. *Addiction history*: Not applicable/applicable

Substance	Type/brand and mode	Quantity/ frequency	Time period	Current use	Dependence
Tobacco					
Alcohol					
Cannabis					
Opium					
Heroin					
Cocaine					
Amphetamine					
LSD					
Solvent					
Intravenous (IV) drug					
Medicine					
Other					
Gambling					
Internet					

Mode of onset:
Impact: Personal/family/social/occupational/legal/other
Comorbid disorders: No/yes
Withdrawal symptoms: No/yes
Treatment received (details):
Comments: In active substance use disorder, a category of dual diagnosis may be made.

12. *Forensic history*: Not applicable/applicable

This is an important part of the psychiatric history as patients with mental health problems have a higher incidence of forensic involvement (Zaman and Makhdum, 2000). It is sometimes difficult to probe forensic history because it is unlikely a patient will tell about his criminal past voluntarily unless asked. A nonjudgmental approach with reaffirming confidentiality may help to elicit forensic history.

Chronologically record the details of all offences, charges, convictions, and sentences passed. It is also important to make mention of any impact this has had on the patient's life and their attitude toward their past. Usual questions to be asked are: *"Have you had any involvement with the law?", "Do you have a police or criminal record?", "Have you ever done anything against the law, or had any allegations made against you?"*

Nature	Yes	No	Number of times	Reason with dates
Police caution				
Arrest				
Conviction				
Ongoing court case/any legal binding/probation?				
Any aggressive behavior/homicidal attempt				

13. *Social history*:

Social situations	Facts and problems/strength and weakness
Social support and network (social contacts—opportunities and functioning)	
Family support and care (living alone or not)	
Accommodation (type, quality, security, sharing, quality of neighborhood)	
Financial situation (source of income, savings, expenditure, debts)	
Domestic activities (daily living skills, daily routine)	
Outdoor activities (travel, holidays, leisure activities)	
Any disadvantageous social condition	

Please note that any positive information on self-harm/addiction/forensic and social history would heavily influence the risk assessment.

14. *History of abuse and violence*: Any childhood abuse (physical, emotional, neglect, or sexual) and violence including details of any domestic violence must be enquired in detail.

■ PREMORBID PERSONALITY

Personality and functioning before the onset of the illness: Briefly describe the nature of personality with regards to patient's general temperament and mood, aspirations, standards, interpersonal relations, social relations, attitude to work, and responsibility. It is difficult to delineate proper personality assessment in a single interview, several extended interviews and discussion with family members may be necessary. Personality consists of enduring characteristics, viz cognition (ways of thinking), affectivity (emotions and feelings), and behavior (interpersonal, reaction, self-control)—some pointers may be identified at the starting interview—general discussion on issues like: Are you happy go lucky, tense, shy, greedy, insecure? Or are you an anxious person? Or evidence of obsessional traits and predominant mood state or the overall quality of relationship with kins, friends, and workmates or some enquiry about hobbies and interests, how was the childhood, religious and moral beliefs, ambitions and aspirations, coping styles, may yield some general impression about premorbid personality.

These are a few clues to understand the basic personality types, but to make a diagnosis of specific disorder, an in-depth review is necessary, and the diagnosis is made from the account after 18 years of age. Behavioral clues of different personality types are tabulated in *Appendix 4: page-68.*

■ CULTURAL HISTORY AND ASSESSMENT
Cultural Issues in Assessment
Cultural Formulation
It provides a systematic method of considering and incorporating sociocultural issues into the clinical formulation *(Appendix 5: page-70).* Cultural assessment improves patient safety in a healthcare organization. Five components of cultural formulation (Focus, 2006; DSM-5, 2013) are:
1. *Cultural identity*: Focus is on ethnicity, migration, age, gender, acculturation, language, socioeconomic status, sexual orientation, religious and spiritual beliefs, disabilities, health literacy, involvement with the culture of origin and host culture.
2. *Cultural explanation of the illness*: The focus is on the patient's explanatory models or idioms of distress, past help-seeking and present treatment expectations and preferences.
3. *Cultural factors related to psychosocial environment and levels of functioning* involve information on available social supports, levels of function or disability, the roles of family systems, religion and spirituality in providing emotional and informational support.
4. *Cultural elements of the relationship between the individual and the clinician* include the ethnocultural identity of physician, language, knowledge about the client's culture, cross-cultural skill and ability and eagerness of the physician to understand client's problem from their cultural context.
5. *Overall cultural assessments*: How the cultural assessment will apply to diagnosis, treatment and care planning?

Cultural history taking: Following is a brief interview format which may be helpful to elicit (by active listening) relevant cultural data for clinical assessment and care (Chowdhury, 2016).

Sl. No.	Cultural issues	Comments/ findings
1	*Ethnocultural identity*	
	Original culture/host culture	
	Mother tongue/present language	
	Immigration/migration history (first/second generation)	
	Level of the tie with original culture	
	The degree of acculturation and level of assimilation with the host culture	
2	*Cultural background*	
	Family role—extended/nuclear family	
	Religious/spiritual beliefs and practices	
	Social support and network	
	Experience of any discrimination and/or prejudice due to race, religion, cultural identity, gender, sexuality, or disability? (stigma)	
	Experience of any trauma, its cultural explanation	
3	*Present problem/difficulties (distress narratives)*	
	Symptoms—culture-specific meanings and its therapeutic implication or culture congruent mood, guilt, somatization, delusion, or hallucination	
	Cultural explanation of cause (EMI) and cure/illness meaning and idioms of distress	
	Past help-seeking(s) (including culture-based)	
4	*Treatment expectations (patient's agenda)*	
	Perception of any cross-cultural barrier or cultural distance?	
	Treatment expectations (what is most helpful?)	
	Involvement of family/community/traditional healer in the treatment process	
	Therapeutic modality desired: Pharmacotherapy/psychotherapy/traditional/ religious/community support	
5	*Cultural formulation*	
	Rate: Level of illness severity/functioning/stressors/social support	
	Diagnosis: Cultural narrative (discuss with the client/family) and medical (discuss and clarify the meanings of diagnostic labels)	
	Note: Any special cultural issues to be addressed in treatment and care Record client's satisfaction score over this assessment	

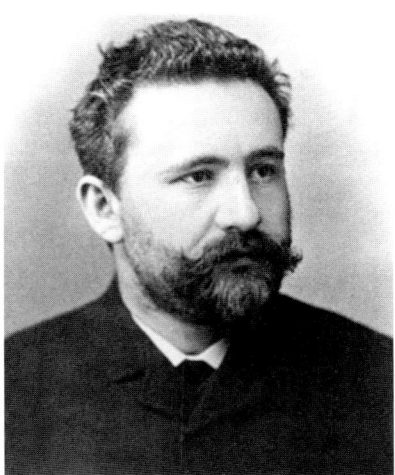

Emil Kraepelin (15.02.1856–7.10.1926), a German psychiatrist, is the founder of modern scientific psychiatry with a profound contribution in psychiatric methodology.

CHAPTER 3

Clinical Examination

■ DEFINITION OF CLINICAL EXAMINATION
- Physical examination
- Central nervous system examination
- Mental state examination

■ PHYSICAL EXAMINATION
- *Physique*: Average/ectomorphic (long and thin muscles/limbs and low-fat storage; usually referred to as slim)/mesomorphic (large bones, solid torso, low-fat levels, wide shoulders with a narrow waist)/endomorphic (increased fat storage; a wide waist and a large bone structure).
- *Handedness*: Right/left
- *General examination*:

Pallor	Lymphadenopathy	Pulse
Cyanosis	Tremors	Blood pressure
Jaundice	Thyroid	Weight
Edema	Skull and spine	Height
Clubbing	Skin	Tobacco smoking

- *Systemic examination*:

Cardiovascular system		
Respiratory system		
Gastrointestinal system		
Endocrinology	Diabetes/obesity	
Genitourinary system		

- Clinical note on physical status and of any positive findings:_____
- Physical diagnosis, if any:_____
- Current investigation/treatment for physical illness, if any:_____

Note: Physical health monitoring in mental health is mandatory. (Please see Appendix 6: page-74)

■ CENTRAL NERVOUS SYSTEM EXAMINATION

1. *Consciousness*: Alert/confusion/clouding/stupor/delirium/coma/other
2. *Speech*: Normal/dysarthric/aphasia/mute
3. *Cranial nerves*:

No.	Name	Test and significance
I	Olfactory	Test smell with a non-noxious agent, especially for head injury (*frontal*)
II	Optic	Visual acuity (*optic nerve, occipital cortex, lens, retina*) and visual fields (*retina, optic nerve, optic chiasma, optic tract, lateral geniculate bodies, optic radiations, occipital lobes*) in each eye separately, both nasal and temporal and superior and inferior. Test for the direct pupillary response
III	Oculomotor	This nerve is responsible for all extraocular movements except down-and-out and abduction. Look for ptosis (drooping of an eyelid) and miosis (small, poorly reactive pupil). Horner's syndrome—ptosis, miosis, and anhidrosis from disruption of sympathetic pathways centrally or peripherally: *midbrain* or *third cranial nerve lesion*.
IV	Trochlear	This nerve moves the eyes down and out (*midbrain*)
V	Trigeminal	This nerve is sensory in three divisions (V1, V2, and V3) to the face. Use the pin/light touch test. Evaluate motor function (muscle of mastication, masseters/pterygoid) and reflexes (afferent of corneal and responsible for jaw jerk) trigeminal neuralgia can occur after herpes zoster infection, and the excruciating pain can lead to suicide
VI	Abducent	Test the patient's abduction of the eyes—diplopia, nystagmus, ocular movement, light reflex, accommodation reflex
VII	Facial	This nerve innervates the muscles of facial expression. Ask the patient to smile and raise eyebrows. If the forehead is involved, the lesion is peripheral; if only the lower face is involved, the lesion is central (*cerebellopontine angle, VIIth nerve*)
VIII	Vestibulocochlear	This nerve is responsible for hearing and vestibulo-ocular reflexes. Whisper multisyllabic words in each year or rub the fingers by each ear with the patient's eyes closed
IX	Glossopharyngeal	This nerve raises the palate and is responsible for the gag reflex. Have the patient open the mouth wide and say "*aah*". The uvula points to the side of the lesion (*medulla*)
X	Vagus	This nerve is responsible and testable for the same functions as cranial nerve IX
XI	Spinal accessory	Ask the patient to shrug his shoulders
XII	Hypoglossal	This nerve is responsible for the motor function of the tongue. Have the patient protrude the tongue out and move it from side to side. The tongue tends to point to the side of the lesion and is slower or weaker in movements on the ipsilateral side of the lesion.

4. *Motor system*:

Issues	Upper Limb		Lower Limb	
	Right	Left	Right	Left
Inspection				
Wasting				
Tone				
Power				
Posture, equilibrium and gait				
Involuntary movement				

- *Muscle wasting*:
  - *Generalized wasting* (malignancy, thyrotoxicosis, myopathies, and motor neurone disease).
  - *Proximal muscle wasting* (muscular dystrophies, syringomyelia, motor neurone disease, inflammatory lesions, myositis)
  - *Peripheral muscle wasting* in forearm [lesion C7-T1, anterior horn cell (poliomyelitis, motor neurone disease, cervical cord tumor), anterior root (cervical spondylosis, cervical tumors), brachial plexus (injury, cervical rib, cervical glandular enlargement, superior pulmonary sulcus tumor), traumatic lesion of radial, median, and ulnar nerve], small muscles of the hand and lower leg or both upper and lower limbs (peroneal muscular atrophy, chronic polyneuritis).
- *Muscle tone:* The degree of tension present in a muscle at rest. Three types of tension:
  i. *Atonic*: Muscle is not used for long periods
  ii. *Hypotonia*: Due to (A) breach in the reflex arc [motor side of the reflex arc (poliomyelitis, polyneuritis, peripheral nerve injury)]; (B) cerebellar disease (ipsilateral hypotonia is common); (C) cerebral or spinal shock after a vascular accident or trauma.
  iii. *Hypertonia*: Three types:
    a. *Clasp-knife spasticity:* Tone is greater in one group of muscles (e.g. quadriceps) than in the antagonists (hamstrings). The resistance is most noticeable when the movement is first made and then is suddenly overcome. Easily demonstrable in elbow and knee. This is a sign of an upper motor neurone lesion and is more marked in the upper limb flexor muscles and the lower limb extensor muscles. Found in upper motor neurone lesions (cerebral thrombosis, hemorrhages, tumor, degenerative diseases, inflammatory lesion and injuries, spinal cord tumors, compressions)
    b. *Lead-pipe rigidity:* There is equal resistance in both agonists and antagonists at any point, i.e. the same degree of hypertonicity is felt throughout each movement. It is a characteristic feature of a lesion of extrapyramidal system, and may be found in upper motor neurone disease.
    c. *Cogwheel rigidity:* Here, the agonists and antagonists contract alternately, rapidly, and regularly during the movement, being marked during the first moments of

testing. Demonstrable nicely at the wrist. Sign of extrapyramidal disease. Found in Parkinsonism, arteriosclerotic degeneration of extrapyramidal system, high dosage of reserpine, chlorpromazine and in carbon monoxide poisoning.

Clonus: Sudden stretching of hypertonic muscle produces reflex repetitive contractions.
- *Muscle power:* Graded system for testing of muscle power: Always compare one side with the other for each muscle at the time it is tested. Test for tone and tremor.
    – 5/5—normal full strength
    – 4/5—against resistance but not fully (may be 4+ or 4)
    – 3/5—against gravity but not resistance
    – 2/5—not against gravity but can move in a plane perpendicular to vector or gravity
    – 1/5—a flicker of contraction but no movement
    – 0/5—no contraction
- *Posture, equilibrium, and gait:* Abnormalities of posture

Akinesia	Intense slowing of the initiation of voluntary movements of limbs and trunk, causing immobility of expression and of posture (Parkinsonism)
Kyphoscoliosis	An abnormal curvature of the spine in both at the coronal and sagittal plane
Lordosis	Inward curvature of a portion of the spine

- *Abnormalities of equilibrium*: Inability to remain upright.

Falling to one side	Vestibular and cerebellar lesion
Falling backwards	Basilar atherosclerosis, basilar invagination, Arnold–Chiari deformity
Falling bizarrely	Hysterical
Romberg's sign	Patient sways from the heels slightly when the eyes are open, but very markedly when the eyes are closed, to the extent that he will fall. Seen in posterior cord compression at a high level, sensory polyneuropathies, subacute combined degeneration of the spinal cord, tabes dorsalis

- *Gait*: Ask the patient to walk in a straight line for at least 10 yards and then return along the same line.

Types	Causes
Dragging the feet	Patient drags 1 foot; upper motor neurone lesion of that leg. *Scissors gait:* In bilateral upper motor neurone lesions, both feet drag and due to spasm of adductor, the legs cross each other and each foot trip up the other. Commonly seen in cerebral diplegia, hereditary spastic paraplegia, advanced cervical spondylosis.
High-stepping gaits	Patient raises the foot too high to overcome a foot drop. The toe hits the ground first. Seen unilaterally in root or peripheral nerve lesions causing anterior tibial muscle paralysis, and bilaterally in polyneuropathies and peroneal muscular atrophy
Shuffling gait	A series of small, flat-footed shuffles. Seen in extrapyramidal disease, cerebral atherosclerosis, Parkinsonism
Ataxic gait	Swings the legs unnecessarily and irregularly, reels to the side of the lesion or ataxia of the trunk, grossly unstable, reels in any direction

Contd...

Contd...

Types	Causes
Waddling gait	The pelvis is rotated through a large arc—congenital dislocation of hips, muscular dystrophy
Hysterical gait	Bizarre, not corresponding to any particular type, varies from moment to moment, does not cause injury and minimized when not observed. *Astasia-abasia*: Inability to stand or walk normally but is able to carry out natural leg movements when sitting or lying down—a symptom of conversion hysteria

- *Involuntary movements:*

Epilepsy and convulsive movements	
Grand mal-epilepsy	Tonic–clonic movements with loss of consciousness
Focal or partial epilepsy	Affect one side or one part of the body only without loss of consciousness
Petit mal-epilepsy	Slight twitching of the eyelids, head nodding, slight jerking of the hands with momentary loss of awareness
Myoclonic jerks	Sudden shock-like contractions of muscle that may occur singly or twice or thrice in rapid succession and may be provoked by touching or by noise
Opisthotonus	State of extreme hyperextension of the neck and spine, varying from arching of the spine to a state of rigidity so great that only heels and vertex touch the bed. May be permanent (meningeal irritation, extrapyramidal rigidity of subacute encephalitis) or spasmodic (tetanus, pontine hemorrhage from tentorial pressure coning, hysteria)
Choreas and dystonias	
Chorea	Hypotonic limbs are flung about in rapid purposeless movements with a flapping of the tongue, hyperextended joints, respiratory/cardiac problems
Athetosis	Slow writhing movements, best seen at wrist, fingers and ankles
Dyskinesias	Dyskinesia is a movement disorder, which consists of effects including diminished voluntary movements and the presence of involuntary movement. Three types: *Acute*—sustained, often painful muscular spasms, producing twisting abnormal postures, usually after parental administration of haloperidol or long-acting fluphenazine, involving the neck, tongue, jaw, oculogyric crisis and rarely opisthotonus. *Chronic*—tardive dyskinesia with prolonged first generation antipsychotics, Levodopa-induced dystonia in Parkinson's disease (PD), and *Nonmotor dystonia*—primary ciliary dyskinesia or biliary dyskinesia
Hemiballismus	Usually involve proximal joints of one arm—wild, rapid, flinging movement of wide radius, occurring constantly, or with a short period of freedom, sufficiently violent to injure the patient or others. Not altered by eye closure, absent during sleep, with increased tone and reflexes of the affected limb. Lesion at subthalamic nucleus or metastatic
Involuntary movements of face and neck	
Facial tics	Stereotyped, repetitive movements such as blinking, screwing up the face or pursing the lips
Perioral tremor	Constant, coarse tremor of orbicularis oris and chin (*GPI*)

Contd...

Contd...

Facial dystonia	Bizarre grimacing of the face with protrusion of tongue (*generalized dystonic state, Huntington's chorea*)
Spasmodic torticollis	Forced turning of the head to one side or even backwards with an elevation of chin and dropping of the occiput.

Tremors: An unintentional, rhythmic, muscle movement involving to-and-fro movements (oscillations) of one or more body parts, most common of all involuntary movements and can affect the hands, arms, head, face, vocal cords, trunk, and legs. Most tremors occur in the hands.

Fine tremor	Thyrotoxicosis
Coarse tremor	Alcoholism, heredofamilial tremor, Parkinsonism, intention tremor
Fine to coarse	Nervousness, anxiety state

5. *Sensory system*: There are two main pathways that relay sensory information:
    i. The dorsal (posterior) column—carries sensory information concerning light touch, vibration, and proprioception
    ii. The spinothalamic tract—carries information concerning pain and temperature.

Basic sensations	Light touch	Pain	Temperature
Proprioceptive sensations	Position sense	Sense of passive movement	Vibration sense
Stereognosis	Ability to recognize an object purely from the feel of its form and texture. Eye closed—each hand one after another—note the accuracy and speed of response. Inability (astereognosis) indicates lesions of the sensory pathway		
Two-point discrimination	Ability to detect that a stimulus consists of two blunt points when they are simultaneously applied. Impairment in parietal lobe lesion		
Graphesthesia	Ability to recognize letters or numbers written on the skin with a blunt point. Impairment (agraphesthesia) in the parietal cortical region		
Test for sensory inattention	The patient is asked to identify when the right side of the body is touched, then the left side and then both sides. Normally, all are identified correctly. With sensory inattention, the patient acknowledges correctly when touched on either side but only identifies one side when both are stimulated together		

6. *Motor-sensory links*:
   Reflexes:

Reflexes	*Right*	*Left*	*Reflexes*	*Right*	*Left*
Biceps			Jaw jerk		
Triceps			Hoffman		
Supinator			Wartenberg		
Knee			Finger flexion		
Ankle			Abdominal		
Patellar clonus			Cremasteric		
Ankle clonus			Planter		

- *Primitive reflexes*: Snout/sucking/palmomental/grasp
  Graded system: Always compare both sides before moving to the next reflex.
  - 0: No reflex
  - 1+: Hyporeflexia
  - 2+: Normal
  - 3+: Hyper-reflexia possibly with unsustained clonus
  - 4+: Marked hyper-reflexia possibly with sustained clonus.
- *Deep tendon reflexes*:
  - *Upper extremities*: Biceps (C5, C6), brachioradialis (C5, C6), triceps (C6, C7), finger flexors (C6-T1)
  - *Lower extremities*: Knee or patellar (L2, 3, 4), ankle (S1, S2)
- *Superficial reflexes*: Abdominal—above the umbilicus (T8, T9, T10) and below the umbilicus (T10, T11, T12). Abdominal (stroke lightly on the abdomen), cremasteric, planter (*Babinski*: Big toe goes up and rest of toes fan out).
  Babinski response: Explain the examination technique to the patient and ask them to relax. Stroke the lateral aspect of the sole of each foot and then come across the ball of the foot medially with a sharp object.
  Normal response: Plantar flexion of the large toe although a response may be difficult to obtain in ticklish individuals where there may be a strong withdrawal.
  Abnormal response: Extension of the large toe, which may be accompanied by fanning of the toes and at time flexion of the knee and hip.
- *Other reflexes*: Finger flexors (hyper-reflexia, if fingers have exaggerated flexion when tapped lightly on the palmar surface); *Hoffman's reflex* (hyperreflexia, if thumb and forefinger flex when flicking the nail of the middle finger); jaw jerk, if exaggerated, will place the lesion at the level of cranial nerve V in the brain stem or above.

  Frontal release signs: Primitive reflexes are often seen, if the frontal lobe is involved; glabellar (with tapping on the forehead, patient cannot stop blinking even if asked); palmomental (stroking palm produces flexion of ipsilateral mentalis muscle); forced grasp (placing fingers between thumb and first finger, patient will grasp); root (patient will move lips to stimulus at corner of mouth); and snout (tapping slightly on lips produces puckering).

  Clonus: It is a series of involuntary muscular contraction due to sudden stretching of the muscle. It is usually associated with upper motor neurone lesions such as in stroke, multiple sclerosis, spinal cord damage, and hepatic encephalopathy. It can be explained as a deep tendon reflex that stems from the abnormality in the neuromuscular activity. Clonus is most common in the ankles, where it is tested by rapidly flexing the foot upward (dorsiflexion). It can also be tested in the knees by rapidly pushing the patella (toward the toes). Wrist clonus is a spasmodic movement of the hand, induced by forcibly extending the hand at the wrist. Only sustained clonus (5 beats or more) is considered abnormal. Clonus appearing after ingesting potent serotonergic drugs strongly predicts imminent serotonin toxicity (serotonin syndrome).

- *Coordination*: Reflects intact motor and sensory systems. Defect points to cerebellar dysfunction or proprioceptive deficiency.

Upper limb: Finger–nose test. (*In cerebellar disease, the arm on the side of the lesion fails, postural ataxia*)	Lower limb: Heel–knee test *(fails in cerebellar disease, sensory ataxia)*
Dysdiadochokinesis: Failure to perform rapidly alternating movements (*cerebellar disease, affected side in motor weaknesses from pyramidal tract lesion*)	Past-pointing test: Sign for both cerebellar and labyrinthine disease

7. *Meningeal signs*:

Neck rigidity	Indicates meningeal irritation from inflammatory and destructive disease of the cervical spine, tonsillar herniation at foramen magnum level. Contraindicates lumbar puncture
Kernig's sign	Limited flexion of each hip and extension of the knee

- Clinical notes on nervous system examination: Summary points
- Central nervous system diagnosis, if any, or need for referral for further neurological assessment:
- Investigation/treatment for CNS diseases, if any:

Note: Please see Appendix 7: page-76.

Quick checkbox for neurological examination

Sl. No.	Test items	Findings/remark
1.	Cranial nerves 1-12	
2.	Motor system	
	Muscle wasting	
	Muscle tone	
	Muscle power	
	Posture	
	Equilibrium	
	Gait	
	Involuntary movement	
3.	Sensory system	
	Touch	
	Pain	
	Temperature	
	Stereognosis	
	2-point discrimination	
	Graphesthesia	
	Sensory inattention	
4.	Motor sensory link	
	Reflexes	
	Coordination	
5.	Meningeal signs	

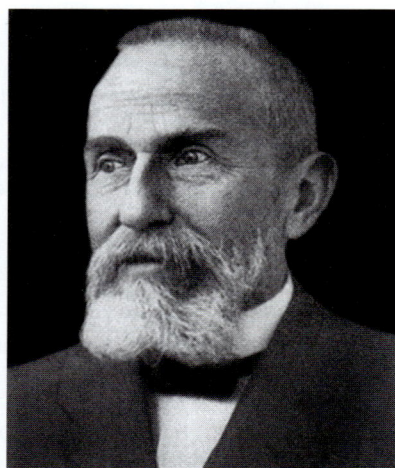

Paul Eugen Bleuler (30.04.1857–15.07.1939), a Swiss psychiatrist who coined the term "Schizophrenia" in 1911 and identified four primary symptoms of schizophrenia, known as Bleuler's "4 A's": Ambivalence, Associative disturbance, Autistic thinking, and Affective incongruity.

■ MENTAL STATE EXAMINATION

This is the most important part of the psychiatric interview. Following is a general frame of interview items that can be followed step by step. A good mental state examination (MSE) reflects the skill and clinical expertise of a psychiatrist. All relevant examination data should be noted in detail because this section is the basis upon which the diagnosis and thus the management of the case depend. The questions should be framed according to the cultural disposition of the patient, and in some situations, the examiner has to apply his or her rational judgment about the grading of impairment of the patient. This section is also very important from the point of judicial reporting. It will be discussed under following headings:

- General appearance and behavior
- Language evaluation
- Voice and speech
- Motor behavior
- Mood and affect
- Examination of thought system
- Examination of perception
- Disorder of identity and will
- Abstract thinking
- Orientation
- Attention and concentration
- Memory
- Constructional ability
- Information and intelligence
- Judgment
- Insight.

General Appearance and Behavior
(Impression at first clinical contact)

The general appearance and behavior can often reflect the inner mental state, and observation can give us a useful insight into the patient's social situation and nature of the emotional state. Basically, three areas need close observation, e.g. physical appearance, activity, and interactions.

1.	The patient is brought	Restrained/Unrestrained		
2.	General look	Well-kempt and tidy/unkempt and untidy/sickly Obese/underweight/overweight/emaciated Overly made up/perplexed and bewildered/drowsy Stuporous/semi-comatose/coma		
3.	Touch with the surrounding	Present	Partial	Absent
4.	Eye contact	Present	Partial	Absent
5.	Hair	Well groomed	Negligent	Disheveled
6.	Finger nails	Appropriate	Negligent and dirty	
7.	Dress	Appropriate	Shabby	Inappropriate
8.	Motor behavior	Appropriate	Inappropriate	
	Underactive/retarded	Hyperactive	Stereotypy	Odd posture
	Waxy flexibility	Ambitendencies	Silly smiling	Echopraxia
	Touching examiner	Negativism	Resistiveness	Aggressive
	Mannerism	Grimaces	Gestures	Tics
	Destructive	Self-injurious	Rigid	Aimless
	Hallucinatory behavior			
9.	Attitude toward examiner/interactions			
	Cooperative	Uncooperative	Attentive	Inattentive
	Exhibitionistic	Frank	Playful	Hostile
	Guarded	Suspicious	Evasive	Seductive
	Attention seeking	Defensive	Indifferent	Eye contact
10.	Rapport	Fully established	Partially established	Not established

Note: Please see Appendix 8: page-78.

Language Evaluation

Handedness		Right/Left	
Spontaneous speech		Not impaired	
Impaired	Output (productivity): normal/abnormal/scant		
Dysarthria	Dysprosody	Aphasia	Paraphasia

Contd...

Contd...

Verbal fluency (flow)	Not impaired				
Impaired:	Hesitant	Stuttering	Muttering	Only when required	Mute
Comprehension	Not impaired			Impaired	
Repetition	Not impaired			Impaired	
Naming and word finding	Not impaired			Impaired	
Reading	Not impaired			Impaired	
Writing	Not impaired			Impaired	
Spelling	Not impaired			Impaired	

- *Test for verbal fluency*: In which the patient has to say as many words as possible from a category in a given time (usually 60 seconds). This category can be semantic, such as animals or fruits, or phonemic, such as words that begin with a particular letter.
  - Overall impression
  - Animal naming test—normal (18–22) animals/60 seconds. Variation ± 5.
  - Score less than 13 in subjects, less than 70 years = Impaired fluency
  - *FAS test*: Assess phonemic fluency—subject has to produce as many words as possible that begin with the letters F, A, and S within 1 minute. Normal 36–60 words; 12 words per letter = reduced fluency.
- *Test for comprehension*:
  - Pointing commands—initially to single object, subsequently to increasing numbers of objects in sequence, normal more than 4.
  - Questions (simple and complex) that require only "yes" or "no" answers, ask at least seven questions (to exclude chance factors).
- *Test for repetition*: Presenting material in ascending order of difficulty, beginning with single monosyllable words, proceeding to complex sentences. Normal persons and brain-damaged subjects without aphasia can accurately repeat sentences of 19 syllables.

Note: Please see Appendix 9: page-80.

Voice and Speech

Patients with psychosis in addition to their dysfunctional thinking process also display disorganized speech. Following is a general guide to assess speech abnormalities.

Volume	Audible		Excessively loud	Abnormally soft	
Tone	Normal fluctuation			Monotonous	
Reaction time			Normal	Delayed	
Rate	Normal		Very slow	Rapid	Pressure of speech

Contd...

Contd...

Flow	Spontaneous	Hesitant	Slurring	Stuttering
	Speaks only on question		Muttering	Mute
Relevance	Relevant		Irrelevant	
Coherence	Coherent		Incoherent	
Goal direction	Goal-directed		Circumstantial	Tangential
Productivity	Normal		Abundant	Scanty
Deviation	Nil		Rhyming	Punning
	Stereotype		Perseveration	Clang association
	Talking past the point			
Word/letter substitution	Phonemic paraphasia	Semantic paraphasia		Neologism
Speech defects	Dysphasia	Dysarthria	Dysphonia	Mutism

Note: Please see Appendix 10: page-82.

Motor Behavior

A careful observation of motor activity should be done. These may include:
- Body posture
- General body movement and gait
- Facial expressions
- *Level of psychomotor activity*: Psychomotor retardation (a general slowing of physical or emotional reactions) is found in depression or negative symptoms of schizophrenia. Psychomotor agitation may occur in anxiety, mania, attention-deficit/hyperactivity disorder (ADHD).
- Presence of dyskinesias like tics or tremors.

    Grossly disorganized behavior may manifest in a variety of ways. People with schizophrenia usually display odd behaviors and have difficulty in formulating and producing goal-directed behavior and activity. Some examples are:
    - Wandering about/talking to themselves/child-like silliness/unpredictable and untriggered agitation, e.g. swearing or shouting/disheveled and malnourished/difficulties with daily activities of living such as preparing meal or maintaining hygiene/unusual dressing like wearing multiple overcoats and gloves on a hot day/inappropriate sexual behavior, e.g. masturbation in public place.

Catatonic features: Completely unaware of the environment, the patient reacts to the environment by either remaining and maintaining a rigid or immobile body posture and resist efforts to be moved or engaging in excessive motor activity.

Note: Please see Appendix 11: page-84.

Mood and Affect

Mood

It is a sustained and pervasive state of emotion. Mood is frequently the reported emotional state.

Mood colors an individual's perception of the environment. Mood is not readily observable, may need to be reported. A particular mood is not necessarily pathological and should be evaluated in the context of the patient's entire history and present mental state examination.

Mood type	Description
Euthymic	Mood in the normal range, which implies the absence of depressed or elevated mood
Sad	Sad, gloomy, sullen, depressed, pessimistic, morose, hopeless
Elevated	An exaggerated feeling of wellbeing—euphoria or elation
Expansive	Lack of restraint in expressing feelings
Ecstasy	Peak state of elation
Anxious	Worried, tense, nervous, apprehensive, frightened, terrified, paranoid
Angry/irritable	Easily annoyed or angered, arrogant, defensive, hostile, furious
Indifferent	Shallow, superficial, cool, distant, apathetic, aloof, affectless
Alexithymia	Inability to feel or describe any sort of mood
Anhedonia	A subjective sense that nothing is pleasurable

Clinical assessment of mood:
1. What is your mood like? (Quality)
2. *Stability (rigid to labile)*: Do you always feel like this?
3. *Reactivity (to external events—none to much)*: Does your mood ever change? When does your mood change?
4. *Intensity (shallow to deep)*: What is the extent or depth of your feeling? On a scale of 0–10, how would you rate your mood? (0 being the worst and 10 being the best)
5. *Periodicity*: Periodic or aperiodic?
6. *Duration*: How long have you felt this way?
7. Whether mood is congruent/incongruent with thought content?

Affect

It is defined as the observable behavior seen in the expression of emotion. Affect responds to change in emotional state (fluctuation). It has three components—facial expression, gestures, and speech. It is expressed through autonomic responses, body movements, alterations in speech and reactive facial expression. Sociocultural norms determine whether an affect is appropriate or abnormal in a particular situation.

Assessment	Normal	Abnormal
Type		Anxious, sad, happy, angry, disgusted, ashamed, detached, or indifferent
Appropriateness	Appropriate, congruent	Inappropriate, incongruent
Intensity	Normal	Blunted/exaggerated/flat/heightened/overly dramatic
Mobility	Mobile	Constricted/fixed/immobile/labile
Range	Full range	Restricted range
Reactivity	Reactive, responsive	Nonreactive, nonresponsive

Note: Please see Appendix 12: page-86.

Examination of Thought System

Thinking refers to the ideational components of mental activity, processes used to imagine, appraise, evaluate, forecast, create, and will. Individuals vary greatly in their predominant cognitive style, i.e. the manner of information processing and decision-making. An obsessional style of thinking is marked by attention to detail and hypervigilance concerning the anticipated implications of a thought or event. A hysterical style of thinking is characterized by global, diffuse, emotionally laden evaluations of the situation without going into details. Thought process may be influenced by stress or fatigue or disease condition.

Clinical evaluation of thought disorder examines four components of thought process, viz. stream, form, possession and content.

1. *Stream (flow)*: It is the speed of the thought, the nature of which may be any of the following:

Normal	Accelerated	Retarded	Mute
Flight of ideas	Pressure of speech	Racing thoughts	Poverty of speech
Thought blocking	Perseveration	Verbigeration	Stereotypy
Incoherence	Word salad	Frequent pauses	Interrupted by cry

2. *Form (continuity)*: Is how thought content is organized to form coherent thoughts and sentences by following the conventional semantic and syntactic rules of language. It may clinically present as:

Circumstantiality	Tangentiality	Derailment	Loosening of association (LOA)	Pressured speech
Flight of ideas	Paragrammatism	Neologism	Echolalia	Palilalia
Thought blocking	Clang association	Illogical thinking	Perseveration	Stereotypy

Formal thought disorders: Mnemonic: NCC DIPTT
- N = *Neologism:* Nonword phonemic combinations used as words.
- C = *Clang association:* A shift in frame of reference driven by a phonetic similarity of words rather than tropical relationships.

- **C = *Circumstantiality:*** Indirect speech, delayed in reaching the point but eventually gets from the original point to the desired goal. The circumstantial style is not necessarily pathologic. Nonpatients circumstantial persons are called "long-winded", found in schizophrenia, dementia, and anxiety disorder.
- **D = *Derailment:*** Gradual or sudden deviation in the train of thought without blocking.
- **I = *Flight of ideas:*** A special case of LOA when there are rapid shifts in the frame of reference and the incoherent associations occur very rapidly. It is not necessarily equivalent to either pressured speech (coherent but rapid speech) or racing thoughts (coherent).
- **P = *Perseveration:*** Inappropriate repetition of words or phrases, seen in dementia, obsessive compulsive disorder (OCD), psychosis.
- **T = *Tangentiality*:** Inability to have goal-directed associations of thought. Found in psychosis and dementia. In dementia, it is also called "rambling".
- **T = *Thought blocking:*** An abrupt interruption in the train of thought before finishing.

Note: Please see Appendix 13: page-91.

3. *Possession:* Alteration in the experience of one's own thought, which may be perceived by the subject as any of the following:

Thought control	Thought insertion	Thought withdrawal	Thought broadcasting	Thought echo
Thought blocking	Referential thinking	Thought diffusion	Magical thinking	Thought alienation

Note: Please see Appendix 14: page-92.

4. *Content:* Also known as belief: Two broad divisions are: (i) nondelusional thoughts, and (ii) delusional thoughts

Nondelusional abnormal thoughts				
Suicidal thought	Homicidal thought	Worthlessness	Hopelessness	Guilt/sin
Obsession	Compulsion	Phobia	Overvalued ideas	Grandiosity
Paranoia	Suspiciousness	Hypochondriasis*	Dysmorphophobia*	Eating disorders*

Note: *Often reach to delusional proportion.

Note: Please see Appendix 15: page-93.

Type of Delusional Thoughts

Delusional thoughts: Delusions are false and firm beliefs not endorsed by the social group, relatively impervious to invalidation. The DSM-IV defines *delusions* as "erroneous beliefs that usually involve a misinterpretation of perceptions or experiences."	
Delusion	According to type: Simple/complex
	According to onset: Primary/secondary
	According to fixity: Complete/partial

Contd...

Contd...

According to span: Systematized/non-systematized

According to the number of content:
Monothematic—that concerns only one particular topic
Poly- or multithematic—where the person has a range of delusions
According to nature of content: Nonbizarre/bizarre

Mood congruent/incongruent: Whether they match with the prevailing mood state?

Delusional experience	Delusional mood		Delusional perception	Delusional memory
Delusional ideas/themes	Persecutory		Reference	Grandiose
	Nihilistic (Cotard's syndrome)	Possession	Hypochondriacal Poverty	Control
	Guilt	Jealousy/Infidelity	Erotic (De Clerambault's syndrome) Infestation (Ekbom's syndrome)	Sin Religious
Delusions of misidentification	Of replacement (Capgras's syndrome)/of disguise (Fregoli's phenomenon)/intermetamorphosis/subjective doubles/mirrored self-misidentification/reduplicative paramnesia/delusional companion/clonal pluralization of self			
Communicated delusions	Folie a deux Folie a trois Folie a famille			Mass delusion

Elicit the nature of delusion:

Simple	Contain few elements
Complex	Contain extensive elaborations of people, motives, and situations
Complete	Held firmly without any doubt
Partial	Have doubts about the delusional beliefs
Systematized	Restricted to well-delineated areas, usually with a clear sensorium and absence of hallucination
Nonsystematized	Extend into many areas of life, new people and situations are constantly incorporated with concurrent mental confusion, hallucination, and affective lability.
Bizarre delusion	When the delusional theme is totally impossible or absurd
Primary (autochthonous)	Instant, without identifiable preceding events—like an unexpected flash of insight, like a bolt from the blue.
• Delusional percept	Interpreting a normal perception with a delusional meaning
• Delusional atmosphere or mood	A strange sense that something uncanny or odd is going on that threatens the patient but in unspecified ways
• Delusional memory	Patient recalls a remembered event or idea that is clearly delusional—here delusion is retrojected in time, often called retrospective delusion
Secondary	Arises out of an underlying mood or from another psychotic phenomenon or from a defect in cognition or perception

Be sure about identifying delusion: Clinically, a delusion is a false belief that is held with absolute passion and conviction that are impervious to reasoning and is out of proportion to the subject's educational, cultural, and social background. Delusions beliefs may be absolutely impossible, simply improbable, or possible but incorrect or without any evidence. Delusions are multidimensional constructs comprising mainly of five dimensions (Combs et al., 2006) as follows: *conviction* (how strongly a belief is held); *preoccupation* (how often the person focuses or thinks about their belief); *pervasiveness* (how widespread and influential the belief is); *negative emotionality* (whether the belief is linked to negative emotional states like anger, depression, or anxiety) and *action-inaction* (whether the belief is linked to behaviors. So, for a belief to qualify as a true delusion, it must have the following features (Kendler et al., 1983).

Conviction	The patient expresses an idea or belief with unusual persistence or force.
Influence or extension	That idea appears to exert an undue influence on his/her life (even to an inexplicable extent).
Pressure	The degree to which the patient is preoccupied and concerned with the expressed delusional beliefs.
Bizarreness	The degree to which the delusional belief departs from culturally determined consensual reality.
Disorganization	The degree to which the delusional beliefs are internally consistent, logical, and systematized.
Secretiveness	Despite his/her total conviction, there is often a quality of secretiveness or suspicion when the patient is questioned about it.
Affective response	The degree to which the patient's emotions are involved with such beliefs.
Reactivity	Any attempt to contradict the belief is likely to arouse an inappropriately strong emotional reaction, often with irritability and hostility.
Odd	The belief is mostly unlikely, and out of keeping with the patient's social, cultural, and religious background.
Deviant behavior	The delusion, if acted out, often leads to behaviors, which are abnormal and/or out of character of the person.
Unusual	Individuals who know the patient will observe that his/her belief and behavior are uncharacteristic and alien.
Not shared by family or community	Sometimes a belief of delusional proportion may be held by a cultural or ethnic group as a part of their world-views.

In a clinical case presentation a rough guide may be presented like:

Content	Delusional thought
Source	How erupted
Evidence	How proved
Conviction	The strength of belief in %
Acting upon	Reaction and what steps taken against the belief

Note: Please see Appendix 16: page-98.

Examination of Perception

Perception: The mental process by which all kinds of data, intellectual, emotional, sensory, and environmental are meaningfully organized.

Imagery: A sensory experience over which the subject has voluntary control and experiences as taking place within the mind. *Apperception*—awareness of the meaning and significance of a particular sensory stimulus as modified by one's own experiences, knowledge, thoughts, and emotions.

The goal of research into perception is to understand how stimuli from the world interact with our sensory systems, forming visual, auditory, tactile, olfactory, and gustatory representations of the world. Research in perception and psychophysics is directed at discovering the lawful relations between environmental events and subjective experience. The modern studies of perception are highly integrative combining cognitive, behavioral, computational, developmental, and neuroscientific approaches. It is thus said that *we do not really see reality, we perceive it.* The understanding of this truth is a fundamental NLP (neuro-linguistic programming) principle.

Clinical evaluation of perceptual disturbances should focus:
- *Which sensory modality is involved*: One (simple hallucination) or multiple (complex hallucination)?
- *Nature of perception*: Intensity, clarity, and frequency.
- *Content of hallucinations*: Personal comments? Commands? Accusatory? Threatening? (narrative should be cited)
- *Location of their sources of origin*: Time of the day—in waking state or while drowsy? Medication?
- *Degree of volitional control over them*: Can they be initiated voluntarily or stopped at will by the patient?
- *Level of conviction (insight) about their reality*: Is the experience factual or product of patient's imagination?
- *Attitude*—pleasant, disturbing, or neutral
- *Nature and degree of influence on the behavior*—patient's reaction: Unbothered? Trying to avoid? Obey commands? Reply or converse with the voices? Attempt to escape?

Disorders of perception:
- *Perceptual distortions*: There is a *real* perceptual object but perceived in a distorted way.
- *Perceptual deceptions*:
  – Illusions
  – Hallucinations
  – Distortions of body image.

Disorders of Perception: Please see Appendix 17: page-104.

Disorder of Identity and Will

(Disintegrated self-experience)

Disorder of will	Catatonic waxy flexibility/echolalia/echopraxia/delusion of passivity
Body image distortion	Anatomy/sensation/perception
Dissociation	Splitting of thoughts/feeling and behavior from everyday integrated conscious awareness
Dissociation of self-experience	Depersonalization/derealization
Dissociative disorder	Changes or disturbances in identity, memory, or consciousness that affect the ability to maintain an integrated sense of self, e.g. amnesia/fuge/dissociative identity disorder
Unawareness of illness	Present/absent

Note: Please see Appendix 18: page-117.

Abstract Thinking

Conceptualization and abstraction: Simple levels of conceptualization are assessed by testing the patient's capacity to discern the similarities and differences between sets of individual words. The capacity to abstract is tested by asking the patient to discern the meaning of well-known metaphorical statements.

Abstract thinking: The ability to appreciate nuances of meaning, multidimensional thinking with the ability to use metaphors and hypothesis appropriately.

Concrete thinking or literal thinking: Limited use of metaphor without understanding nuances of meaning—one-dimensional thought.

    How to test abstract thinking?

Response to proverb	Use popular proverb and note the explanation/interpretation
Similarities and differences	Use simple object or animal test
Conceptual series completion	Solve unfamiliar and complex verbal problems

Proverb test: Examines the degree of abstraction demonstrated by the patient in the interpretation of the proverb. At least three proverbs should be given, read each proverb as written, do not paraphrase or otherwise explain the proverb. Rate each response as abstract—2 points; semi-abstract—1 point, and concrete—0 points. A concrete response or an absence of any abstract responses should suggest an impairment of abstract ability.

Test items:
- A drowning man will clutch at a straw
- Rome was not built in a day
- Little learning is a dangerous thing.
  Scoring: A drowning man will clutch at a straw.
  0—concrete: "Do not let go when you are in the water".
  1—semi-abstract: "It is a last resort".
  2—abstract: "A person in trouble will try anything to get out of it."

- *Similarities:* In verbal similarities test, the patient should explain the basic similarity between two overtly different objects or situations, and it requires analysis of the relationship, the formation of verbal concepts, and logical thinking.
  Test items: "Please tell me how they are similar or alike".
  1. Potato: Cauliflower
  2. Lotus: Rose
  3. Cow: Goat
  4. Motorcar: Airplane
  5. Horse: Apple
  Scoring: Potato—cauliflower
  2 points = Vegetables
  1 point = Food, they grow in the ground, edible
  0 points = Buy in the market
- *Conceptual series completion*: Instruction—"I am going to show you some numbers, letters, or words in series. Each series will be incomplete and needs an additional word, letter, or number to complete it each dash (-) calls for that missing number or word or letter".
  Test items:
  Series correct response:
  1. ABCD____   E
  2. 1, 4, 7, 10,____   13
  3. AZ, BY, CX, D____   W
  4. Lotus-Mango-Rose-Coconut-Sunflower-Date-Tulip-___   Any fruit

Note:
- *Autistic thinking:* Preoccupation with inner thoughts, daydreams, fantasies, private logic; egocentric, subjective thinking lacking objectivity, and connection with external reality.
- *Dereistic thinking:* Thinking not in accordance with the facts of reality and experience and following illogical, idiosyncratic reasoning.

Orientation

It is the ability to comprehend and interpret the imminent environment. Accurate orientation requires the integrity of attention, perception, memory, and ideation. Orientation to time is generally the first function lost and usually indicates early or mild brain damage. Orientation to place is often lost next. Last, in cases with the most severe damage, a person does not know who he or she is.
Test items:

Time	Place	Person
Day	Floor	Accompanying relative
Date	Building	Another person, if present in the room
Month	Place	
Year	City/State/Country	

Note: Disorientation: The lack of being able to correctly identify oneself, one's location, or the date and time, is a sign of altered mental status, i.e. when the sensorium is clouded, as in torpor, obtundation, dreamy states, delirium, or fugue. Disorientation for time and place usually indicates organic brain disorder like dementia, delirium, acute confusional state, partial seizure, brain tumors, and intoxication. Disorientation for personal identity is rare and is associated with psychogenic or postictal fugue states, other dissociative disorders, and agnosia (loss of the ability to recognize sensory inputs). It may occur in panic attacks, post-traumatic stress disorder (PTSD) and acute psychotic state.

Attention and Concentration

Attention refers to the ability to attend to a specific stimulus, without being distracted by external or internal stimuli.

Test for attention: Digit repetition test: Repeat digit at a rate of one per second. Check for correct digit repetition.

Test digits	Check
3 -7	
7 -4 -9	
8 -5 -2 -7	
2 -9 -6 -8 -3	
5 -7 -2 -9 -4 -6	
8 -1 -5 -9 -3 -6 -2	
3 -9 -8 -2 – 5 -1 -4 -7	
7 -2 -8 -5 -4 -6 -7 -3 -9	

Intact/impaired: Patient of average intelligence can accurately repeat 5 to 7 digits without difficulty. In a nonretarded patient without obvious aphasia, inability to repeat more than 5 digits indicates defective attention.

Concentration or vigilance is the ability to sustain attention over an extended period. Ability to concentrate depends on: commitment, enthusiasm for the task, skill at doing the task, emotional and physical state and on the current environment.

Test for concentration: Digit scan test: Repeat letters at a rate of one per second. The subject has to indicate by tapping the table whenever he or she hears the letter "A" or aa.

L	T	P	E	A	O	A	I	C	T	D	A	L	A	A
A	N	I	A	B	F	S	A	M	R	Z	E	O	A	D
P	A	K	L	A	U	C	J	T	O	E	A	B	A	A
Z	Y	F	M	U	S	A	H	E	V	A	A	R	A	T

Intact/impaired:
Currently, only preliminary standardized norms exist for this test. An average person should complete the task without error (mean 0.2); a sample of randomly selected brain-damaged patients made an average of 10 errors. Examples of common organic errors are:
- Failure to indicate when the target letter has been presented (omission error)
- Indication made when a nontargeted letter has been presented (commission error).
- Failure to stop tapping with the presentation of subsequent nontargeted letters (perseveration error).

Note: Please see Appendix 19: page-120.

Memory

Definition: It is a process whereby what is experienced or learned is established as a record in the central nervous system (*registration*); where it persists with a variable degree of performance (*repetition*) and can be recollected or retrieved from storage at will (*recall*). Clinically, memory is subdivided into three basic types based on the time span between stimulus presentation and memory retrieved.
- *Immediate memory or immediate recall:* Reproduction, recognition or recall of perceived material within seconds after the presentation.
    Question asked: Digit repetition test or digit span test. Both forward and backward span.
    – Examiner verbally presents a series of digits asking the patient to listen carefully, so that he/she can repeat them.
    – Digits are presented slowly, at a rate of one digit per second distinctly without grouping or pairing them.
    – Numbers should be presented randomly without natural sequences. The patient is asked to repeat the digit series.
    – Later, a new series of digits given and asked to repeat them in reverse order.
    Scoring—with a patient of average intelligence 5-6 digits forwards/3-4 digits backwards—is adequate.
    Test items (forward): Intact/impaired

Test digits	Check
3 -7	
7 -4 -9	
8 -5 -2 -7	
2 -9 -6 -8 -3	
5 -7 -2 -9 -4 -6	
8 -1 -5 -9 -3 -6 -2	
3 -9 -8 -2 – 5 -1 -4 -7	
7 -2 -8 -5 -4 -6 -7 -3 -9	

Test item (backward): Intact/impaired

Test digits	Check
9 -2	
1 -7 -4	
5 -2 -9 -7	
6 -8 -3 -5 -1	
2 -9 -4 -7 -3 -8	
4 -1 -9 -2 -2 -5 -1	
8 -5 -3 -9 -1 -6 -2 -7	
2 -1 -9 -7 -3 -5 -8 -4 -6	

- *Recent memory:* Recall of events over the past 2 days. It refers to the patient's capacity to remember current, day-to-day events.

  Tests:
  – Ask the patient to recall and describe some events of the past 24 hours.
  – Give the patient three unrelated words—an object, a color, and an address—ask him to remember this information. He/she is asked to recall it after 5–10 minutes.
  – The following questions can be asked:
     • Where do you live?
     • What is the date today?
     • What is your address?
     • What is the day of the week?
     • What is the season?
     • What are the names of other people who live with you?
     • When did you come to the hospital?
     • With whom did you come?
     • How did you come? Detailed mode of transport.
     • When have you eaten this morning?

  Score: Normal people perform perfectly (performance correlates with education level)

- *Remote memory:* Refers to the recollection of facts or events in distant past, i.e. events that occurred in the past.

Questions asked:
1. *Personal information*:
   • Birthplace; about schooling; occupation, place of work, time of work
   • Family information like wife's/children's name; the age of wife or children; mother's maiden name
2. Historical facts: Local, regional, or historical events, known to have occurred during the patient's lifetime, which any person in the community with the same sociocultural background would ordinarily know.

Note: Please see Appendix 20: page-121.

Constructional Ability

Constructional ability or praxis: Capacity to draw or construct two- or three-dimensional figures or shapes. This nonverbal cognitive function is a very complex perceptual motor task that involves integration of occipital, parietal, and frontal lobe functions.

A disturbance in praxis (apraxia) is suggestive of organic brain disease. This ability tests the following: (1) accurate visual perception, (2) integration of perception into kinesthetic images, (3) translation of kinesthetic images into the final motor patterns necessary for the construction, and (4) limb strength and coordination.

Tests: Usual clinical tests (Strub and Black, 1995) are:
- *Reproduction drawings:* The drawings presented here may be given to the patient with the instruction: "Please draw this design exactly as it looks to you". Abnormalities may be rotation, perseveration, or "closing in".
- *Drawings to command:* Patient is asked to draw three pictures as asked: (1) a clock with the numbers and hands; (2) a flower in a flowerpot; and (3) a house in perspective, so that you can see two sides and the roof.

Scoring:
- 0—poor: Nonrecognizable reproductions or gross distortion
- 1—fair: Moderate distortion, and
- 2—good: minimal distortions with adequate integration.

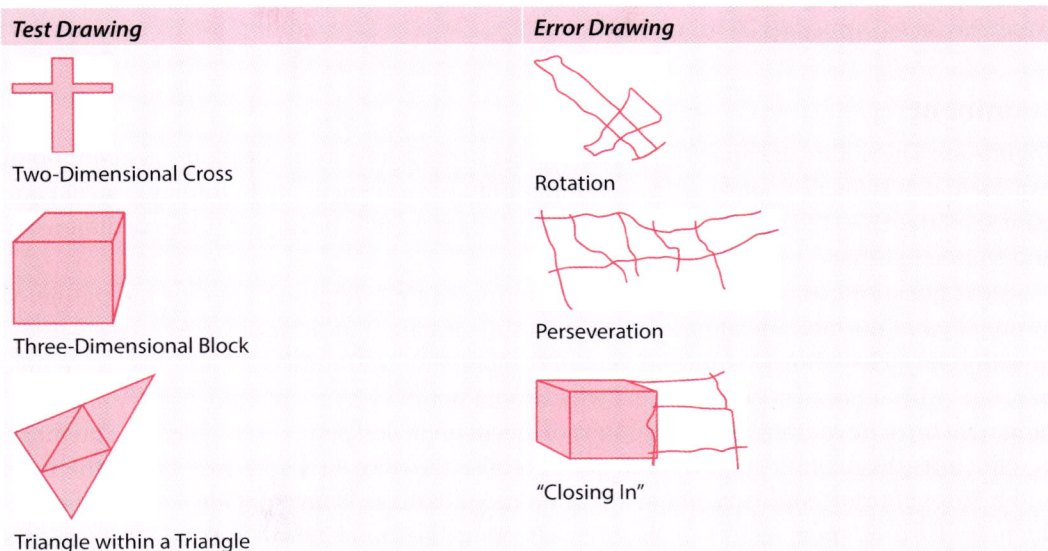

Information and Intelligence

Ask appropriate questions according to culture and educational standard of the patient, which can offer you a reasonable estimate of patient's store of knowledge, fund of general information, and intelligence level.

Areas	Comments: Poor/average/above average			
Comprehension	There are no tests for comprehension. It is evaluated as the interview proceeds. It is evaluated by his or her grasp of the importance of the immediate situation: Does the patient know why he or she is at this clinic? Does the patient appreciate that he or she is ill or in need of treatment? Does the patient understand the purpose of the examination?			
Vocabulary	Grade school level, high school level, fluent, consistent with education			
Counting	Add these numbers: (15 + 12 + 7) or multiply these numbers: (25 × 6)			
Calculation	"If a kilogram of potato costs 18 rupees and you give the cashier a hundred rupee note, how much change should you get back?"			
General knowledge	Name the current president/name four of the largest cities in the country			
Level of formal education				
Level of self-education				
Intelligence*	Average		Above average	
Subnormal	Mild	Moderate	Severe	Profound

Note: *Supplemented by IQ test

Note: Please see Appendix 21: page-125.

Judgment

Definition: The ability or capacity to draw correct conclusions from the material acquired by experience. It reflects a complex mental functioning involving analytic thinking, social and ethical tendencies, and depth of understanding. Judgment may be impaired in one dimension and spared in others.

Most questions about judgment center on topics that demonstrate that the patient is aware of what normal, social interaction or responses are. For example, a frequently asked question is: "what should you do if you are in a theater and notice a fire?" An alternative may be: "why are laws necessary?" or "why should people stay away from a bad company?" Judgment must be examined in the context of recent behavior, patient's intelligence, memory, and the integrity of other cognitive functions, as also the diagnosis and treatment adherence and history of prior impulsive behavior. Impaired judgment is not specific to any diagnosis but may be a prominent feature of disorders affecting the frontal lobe of the brain. If a person's judgment is impaired due to mental illness, there may be a concern for the person's safety or the safety of others.

Three types of judgment are:

Areas	Examination	Satisfactory	Impaired
1. Personal	The ability for a sufficiently realistic future plan in the context of education, job, or life situation		
2. Social	The ability for a realistic explanation of social events or situations		
3. Test	*Response to an imaginary situation (e.g. stamped postcard* or fire breakout story)*: May by *critical* (answers critically with detailed elaboration) or *reflexive or automatic* (instantaneous action response)		

Note: *"What would you do if you found a stamped, addressed envelope lying in the street?"

Insight

Definition: Subject's degree of awareness and understanding about being ill. The term "insight" has many meanings, but for psychiatric interview, it implies five dimensions (Amador and David, 1998): (1) awareness of mental illness, (2) awareness of specific signs and symptoms of the disorder; (3) attribution of symptoms to the disorder; (4) understanding the social consequence of the disorder; and (5) awareness of the need of medical treatment.

Insight may be measured in terms of the patient's understanding of his or her health condition as being primarily either psychological or medical condition. Insight has a deep influence on assessment as well as on treatment compliance. Complete lack of insight is often seen in psychotic disorders or dementia and is an important consideration in treatment planning and in assessing the capacity to consent to treatment. Poor insight is common in schizophrenia. Approximately, one-half of all patients exhibit severe, pervasive, and persistent problems with insight. Poor insight has a strong correlation with noncompliance and thus the effectiveness of treatment (Amador and Gorman, 1998). Poor insight might also indicate a diagnosis of a personality disorder or low intelligence.

Grade I	Complete denial of illness
Grade II	Slight awareness of being sick but denying it at the same time
Grade III	Awareness of being sick but blaming it on external factors
Grade IV	Awareness that illness is due to something unknown to/in the patient
Grade V	*Intellectual insight*: The admission that the patient is ill and the symptoms or failure in social adjustments are due to the patient's own particular irrational feelings or disturbances without applying this knowledge to future experiences.
Grade VI	*True emotional insight*: Emotional awareness of the motives and feelings within the patient and the important persons in his/her life, which can lead to basic changes in behavior

Insight is complex and multidimensional. Insight is not an all or none phenomenon, and there are degrees of insight. Insight is subjective, and the reason for assessing this is to examine whether the patient and the psychiatrist share the same ideas about what is wrong and what to do about it (treatment). Psychiatric illnesses in which the patient has an altered sense of reality can affect insight. The patients understanding of their condition and their perceived need for treatment can vary from day to day and hour to hour. Remember, insight fluctuates and can be present in a variable measure. Cultural factors may influence insight. Lack of insight can lead to risky behavior.

Summary points of Mental State Examination:

Item	Descriptor
General appearance and behavior (GAB)	
• Appearance	Posture, clothing, grooming, hygiene
• Behavior	• Facial expression, eye contact, rapport and engagement, anxious/calm/agitated/aggressive, psychomotor activity/hyperactivity/hypoactivity, tremors, repetitive or involuntary movements, mannerisms • Attitude toward the assessment—cooperative, suspicious, hostile, perplexed
Speech	Rate (rapid, pressured), volume (normal, soft, loud), tonality (monotonous, tremulous), quantity (normal, minimal, voluble), quality (accent, rhythm, impediments)
Affect (patient's observable emotions)	• Range (restricted, blunted, flat, expansive) • Appropriateness (inappropriate, incongruous) • Stability (stable, labile)
Mood	
• *Subjective* (how patient tells you it is)	Depression, anxiety, mania
• *Objective* (do emotions appear appropriate to the pathology)	
Thought	
• Stream	Pressured speech, flight of ideas, poverty of speech
• Form (FTD)	Thought blocking, racing thoughts, logical connection, flight of ideas, loosening of association
• Possession	Thought control, thought blocking, referential thinking
• Content	Preoccupations, overvalued ideas, delusions, ideas of reference, obsessions, compulsions, suicidal, homicidal
Perception	Hallucinations, illusions, heightened perception, dissociative symptoms (derealization/depersonalization)
Cognition	
• Level of consciousness	Alert, drowsy, intoxicated, stuporous
• Orientation	To time, place, person
• Memory	Immediate, short-term (recent), and long-term (remote)
• Attention and concentration	Mini-Cog or MMSE may help
• Visuospatial processing	
• Language functions	
	Level of distractibility, subtract serial 7's—counting backwards from 100/spell "WORLD" forward and backward

Contd...

Contd...

• General knowledge • Abstract thinking/reasoning	Constructional ability (copying diagram or face of a clock)
	Naming objects, reading, writing, following instructions
	Historical/current affairs
	Describing conceptual similarity between two things, explaining proverbs
Judgment (ability to accurately assess a situation and act appropriately in response)	Intact or impaired
Insight (an individual's awareness of their illness and its effects and implications)	Good, partial, or poor

After completing the mental state examination, the following clinical issues have to be addressed:
- Any investigations indicated (psychological, neurological, radiological, or laboratory tests)
- Extended interview intended (with family members or other agencies)
- Diagnostic formulation with differential diagnosis
- Treatment/care plan including risk assessment and management/referral
- Summary findings and follow-up monitoring.

The next section will cover these issues.

Chapter 4

Additional Evaluation, Management and Related Issues

> **This chapter will be discussed under following headings:**
> - Risk Assessment
> - Mental Capacity Assessment
> - Case Formulation
> - Treatment/Care Plan
> - Safeguarding
> - Case Summary
> - Clinical Record
> - Safe Prescribing

■ RISK ASSESSMENT

Predictability of human behavior is always difficult. Risk has a dynamic potential and depends upon an interplay between an individual's personality pattern, features of their illness (and treatment compliance), and the specific ongoing life situations. Risk assessment is a clinical process of critically weighing objective and subjective factors at a particular point of time. Good clinical practice is to make a reasonable assessment of one's risk to him and others, collate all available information, and communicate this to appropriate person or agencies, so that suitable measures can be planned adequately beforehand. Following is a broad format that may help to collect information on major risk factors:

Risk factors	Past history (historical) No/yes—specify	Current (date) No/yes—specify
Risk of deliberate Self-harm (suicide)	• How many times—when • Method • Use weapon • Outcome • Family history of suicide	• Current SH/suicidal thoughts • How frequent? • Intent—Weak/strong? • Plan (passive/active)?

Contd...

Contd...

Risk of violence/harm to others	• Nature • Method • Use weapon • Outcome • How many times	• Ideas/thoughts or plan • Verbally expressed any target
Risk of self-neglect (health + hygiene + compliance)	• Health • Hygiene • Compliance • Staying alone/lack of social relationship	
Risk of abuse and exploitation from others	• Physical • Emotional • Economical • Sexual	
Misuse of drugs/alcohol	• Type • Method • Outcome	Current active use?
Psychotic symptoms	• Persecutory delusion • Delusion of jealousy • Delusion of guilt • Nihilistic delusion • Command hallucination	
Significant forensic history	• Nature • Outcome	
Significant stress	• Life issues (marital, bereavement, job, etc.) • Physical illness • Level of distress	
Present diagnosis		
Any protective factor in mitigating the risk		
Current risk potentials with points in favor	• No risk • Low-to-medium risk • High risk	

Risk Management

First define the risk and then plan the management to reduce the risk by appropriate intervention (Goldberg and Murray, 2007).

First step: From the historical facts and the current state of the patient:
- Define the *risk behavior* and estimate the *seriousness* of the potential harm
- Estimate the *probability* that the risk will become reality
- Estimate the *imminence* that the risk will become reality
- Estimate any *protective factors* present

The *risk management plan* should address the following issues:
1. How serious is the risk?
2. Is the risk specific or general?
3. How immediate is the risk?
4. How volatile is the risk?
5. What specific treatment and interventions can best reduce the risk?
6. What plan of management is needed to reduce the risk?
7. What are the protective factors?

Risk management may be a short- or long-term process and involves continuous feedback monitoring from the professional team. Responsibilities should be distributed among the team members or other agencies and to be reviewed (both success and failures) periodically. For each patient, the risk management plan would be different as per his/her risk presentation and each step should be properly documented in writing and should be communicated to all the concerned team/professional members.

The document on "Risk Assessment and Risk Management in Psychiatric Practice" by Morgan (2007), available at Royal College of Psychiatrists website, is very helpful in this regard.

Note: Risk Factors for Violence in Psychosis: Please see Appendix 22: page-126.

■ MENTAL CAPACITY ASSESSMENT

Mental capacity assessment of the patient, either for treatment negotiation or for research purpose, is a legal safeguard for the health professionals (Jacob and Chowdhury, 2009). At the end of the treatment plan or summary, it is a good practice to note: *"the patient has full capacity for the decision of treatment choice and consented for the present treatment plan"*. If the patient lacks such capacity then the assessment of mental capacity has to be undertaken and should be documented. Mental capacity is a legal concept related to the ability to enter into a valid contract. In England and Wales, the Mental Capacity Act (2005) provides a statutory framework to protect vulnerable people who are not able to make their own decisions. The Act has five key principles (Singhal et al., 2008):
1. A presumption of capacity
2. The right for individuals to be supported to make their own decisions
3. The right for individuals to make what might be seen as eccentric or unwise decisions
4. Anything done for or on behalf of people without capacity must be in their best interests
5. The least restrictive intervention must be used.

The Act sets out a test for mental capacity assessment, which is both "decision specific" and "time specific". No one can be labeled "incapable" simply as a result of a particular medical condition or diagnosis (DOH, 2005).

Assessment of Capacity for an Adult Patient

(*Adapted from DOH Guideline, 2008*)

Step A: Details of the decision (e.g. treatment plan/ECT/change of accommodation or care facilities, etc.)

Step B:
1. Patient has an impairment of, or disturbance in, the functioning of his/her mind or brain;
2. The patient is unable to make the decision for himself/herself; in as much as:
    - The patient is unable to understand the information relevant to the decision
    - The patient is unable to retain that information
    - The patient is unable to use or weigh that information in the decision-making process; or
    - The patient is unable to communicate his/her decision by any means *(e.g. if in a coma, or "locked-in syndrome")*

If both parts (1 and 2) of the above test are met, then the patient is assessed to lack capacity in relation to this decision.

Step C: If there is no valid and applicable advance decision; nor any personal welfare attorney, or appointed deputy, the responsible health professional, caring for the patient should make the decision, which she/he believes to be in the patient's best interests.

Step D: In making the decision on behalf of the patient who lacks capacity, to determine what is in the *best interests* of the patient, the following steps should be taken:
- Pros and cons of the rationality and urgency of the proposed treatment
- Consider the patient's past and present wishes and feelings, beliefs and values, and the risks and benefits of what is proposed, and any alternative (s)
- Consulting others involved in the treatment process including any legal representative, if appointed for the patient
- Details of the decision proposed.

(*Best interests:* A patient's best interests are not limited to their best medical interests. Other factors, which form part of the best interests' decision, include the wishes and beliefs of the patient when competent, their current wishes, their general well-being and their spiritual and religious welfare.)

■ CASE FORMULATION

The standard format advocated by Oxford Handbook of Psychiatry (2013) is quite simple and useful. A slightly modified version may be used as follows:
- *A brief synopsis of the case*: Summary of the salient points elicited in the psychiatric assessment such as:
    - Demographic data
    - Previous psychiatric diagnosis/treatment
    - Positive medical history of significance
    - Description of current symptoms (presenting problem with onset)
    - Positive findings from Mental State Examination (MSE) (use labels for psychopathological findings such as "delusion of guilt" or "third person auditory hallucination")
    - Risk assessment (harm to self-suicide/harm to others—violence)
    - Patient's Explanatory Model of Illness (EMI) and any significant cultural issues.

- *Working diagnosis*: On the basis of all these: *provisional diagnosis* (if you need more information or wish to investigate more, which is not possible right now) or *diagnosis (may be the solitary or dual diagnosis)*.
- *Differential diagnosis*: List, in order of probability, two or three diagnoses that should be considered here and should be investigated. Give the evidence for and against each diagnosis that you consider in differential diagnosis.
- *Formulation*: Here is the focus on etiological factors, namely the three Ps: *predisposing, precipitating,* and *perpetuating* factors for the current illness.

Kuruvilla and Kuruvilla (2010) have provided this useful format for formulation:
- Biological factors (e.g. genetic, physical illness, drugs)
- Psychological factors (e.g. obsessive personality traits)
- Sociological factors (e.g. poor social support, unemployment)
- Predisposing factors (e.g. family history of mood disorder)
- Precipitating factors (e.g. childbirth)
- Perpetuating factors (e.g. husband's alcohol abuse).

Psychodynamic Formulation

Mace and Binyon (2005) defined psychodynamic case formulation as *"A psychodynamic formulation should summarize the dynamics of a clinical situation, allowing its apparent motivation to be grasped by someone who is otherwise unfamiliar with it. The formulation will explain the nature and timing of key developments up to the present and will facilitate predictions of what is likely to happen in the future. It incorporates a summary of relevant background information, alongside a series of systematic inferences drawn from this. As a clinical report, it must account for symptoms and disabilities in the light of adverse events and developmental patterns. As a psychodynamic explanation, it will discuss interpersonal and intrapsychic mechanisms. It is therefore likely to refer to internal conflict, developmental difficulties, or unconscious processes."*

They proposed four levels of a psychodynamic formulation as:
1. Recognizing the psychological dimension
2. Constructing an illness narrative
3. Modeling a formulation
4. Naming the elements.

■ TREATMENT/CARE PLAN

A good and concise treatment plan should include the following issues:
- Any diagnostic laboratory investigation or psychological tests planned
- Any extended interview either with the patient or other significant person intended
- Plans of treatment as ambulatory or inpatient (immediate and long-term)
- Plans for medication and care plan, if needed appointment of key worker
- Plans for psychological or other therapy, if any
- Referrals to other disciplines, if needed

- Date and time of next follow-up visit with a detailed written care plan
- Detailed planning on risk management, involving the patient, any other health professionals or person or any agencies.

It is important to note that the patient is an important partner in the planning of treatment schedule. The more one involves the patient in planning treatment, the more likely that he/she will follow through with the plan.

Note: The detailed risk–benefits of medication or treatment procedure should be thoroughly discussed with the patient with drug information leaflets, and his agreement should be recorded in the clinical note.

Referral: In many cases, specialist opinion and advice are necessary, either because of comorbidity or of the special nature of the clinical problem. In adult mental health, the usual referrals are for:

Substance use or alcohol problems	Eating disorders	Forensic problems
Neuropsychiatry problems	Learning disability	Personality disorders
Psychotherapy	Cognitive-behavioral therapy	Sexual, marital, or couple therapy

Please note that all decisions should be taken in consultation with the patient. If the patient lacks "capacity to consent" then the decisions should be discussed and taken in an appropriate forum like next of kin or best interest meeting or professional meeting involving all concerned in the context of the legal framework.

Compliance describes a good follow-up, but now the term is being replaced with adherence, which implies less passivity. A patient chooses to adhere, while he is made to comply. Lazare et al. (1975) have outlined a useful approach to negotiate a treatment plan with the patient. The usual steps are:

- Elicit the patient's agenda
- Negotiate a mutually agreed treatment goal
- Explain to the patient what you intend to do and why
- *Fostering a therapeutic alliance*: By providing treatment with respect/fully informed/confidence building for good compliance.
- Implement the agreed-on plan with medication trial and follow-up appointments.

It is a good medical practice to offer a detailed written care plan with a detailed prescription of medications to the patient, with a copy to his/her general practitioner (GP) or referral doctor.

■ SAFEGUARDING

What and Why Safeguarding?

Safeguarding means protecting people's health, well-being and human rights, and allowing them to live a free and dignified life free from harm, abuse and neglect. It is a fundamental concern of Mental Health Law and ethics (Mandelstan, 2009).

People with care and support such as children, older people, people with disabilities, and people with communication difficulties or with cognitive impairment are vulnerable to be abused and neglected. So according to the abuse situation, a potentially *vulnerable child* or a *vulnerable adult* should be identified during the course of assessment and accordingly necessary steps for child protection or safeguarding adult or older people should be called for.

What is a vulnerable adult? A vulnerable adult is a patient who is or may for any reason unable to take care of him-/herself or unable to protect against significant harm or abuse and exploitation.

All health professionals should be aware of the different types of abuse and should take appropriate steps to protect the person. Following is a brief list of abuse:
- Physical abuse
- Domestic violence or abuse
- Sexual abuse
- Psychological or emotional abuse
- Financial or material abuse
- Modern slavery (human trafficking; forced labor; domestic servitude; sexual exploitation; debt bondage)
- Discriminatory abuse
- Organizational/institutional abuse
- Neglect and acts of omission
- Self-neglect.

■ CASE SUMMARY

The summary: A concise description of all the important aspects of the case to grasp the essential features of the problem and would be an essential document in follow-up. The formulation is an assessment of the case. The usual format should cover the flowing:
- Identification data
- Reason for referral and referrer
- Family history
- Personal history
- Past medical/psychiatric history
- Premorbid personality
- Physical examination
- Mental state examination
- Investigations
- Final diagnosis with International Classification of Diseases (ICD)/Diagnostic and Statistical Manual of Mental Disorders (DSM) code
- Treatment and response
- Notes on prognosis
- Conditions for discharge (if admitted)
- Risk management plan.

This is an important document frequently needed for follow-up monitoring of cases or transfer of the case to other professional agencies.

■ CLINICAL RECORD

A good clinical record should be clear, objective, and professionally accurate, clinically sound and maintain the medicolegal aspect, if necessary. Although the doctors are not above making mistakes they should and must exercise a reasonable standard of skill and care in their deliberations at all times.

Keeping a good clinical record is not only a very important skill but also provides good legal safeguarding. Few things to be aware of:
- Always date and sign your clinical notes.
- If you want to change then add an amendment.
- Any correction should be properly signed with the date.
- All recorded clinical materials are confidential. GMC (2017) states that "The duty of confidentiality goes beyond undertaking not to divulge confidential information; it includes a responsibility to make sure that written patient information is kept securely".

A good clinical record should have the following content:
- History of current and past illness
- Examination findings: Both positive and relevant negative, any objective measurement [blood pressure (BP)/pulse/weight, etc.]
- Differential diagnosis
- Investigations—with results
- Referral—any opinion given
- *Patient information*: Information given to patient regarding risk-benefits of proposed treatment/investigation
- Consent
- Capacity
- Treatment—details of medications with doses and justification
- Follow-up plan
- *Progress*: An outline of virtual progress
- Do not write any offensive comments, e.g. racist, sexist, or ageist remarks on the note.

■ SAFE PRESCRIBING

Prescribing faults and prescription errors are major problems among medication errors (Velo and Minuz, 2009). A prescription error is often a serious mistake in medicine. An utmost caution should be exercised in writing a prescription as follows:
- Be sure the identity of the patient is correct on the prescription (name/date of birth/address, etc.)
- Always consult national formulary before writing a medication.
- The script should be legible and understandable, special care in writing the drug name (generic name is preferred to avoid confusion with different trade names)—signed with the date.
- Most common medication errors are—wrong name/wrong drug/wrong dose, and wrong frequency.
- Appropriate indications must be fulfilled.

- Drug combinations—rationality to be justified
- Polypharmacy should be avoided, and, if necessary, it should be justified and evidence based
- Adverse effects—warned the patient about more common side effects
- Drug interactions—aware/knowledge
- *Duration of treatment*: Clearly spelt and written
- *Consumer information*: By leaflet, may be handed over to the patient
- "When required" (PRN) drug treatment should be clearly spelt and written
- *Dose*: The aim is to find the minimum effective dose. For prescribing to children or older people more precautions and check should be exercised. Dosage should be written in a clear and unambiguous way, with the frequency and route of administration, avoiding abbreviations and put a 0 before decimal points—0.2 mg.
- Keep a copy of the prescription in the patient's clinical record.
- Recently, many health providers have computerized electronic-prescription system. Be familiar with the system.

Section 2

Appendices

1. History of Present Complaints
2. Genogram
3. Premenstrual Syndrome
4. Premorbid Personality
5. Cultural Assessment in Psychiatry
6. Physical Health Monitoring in Mental Health
7. Central Nervous System Examination
8. General Appearance and Behavior
9. Language Evaluation
10. Voice and Speech
11. Catatonia
12. Mood and Affect
13. Formal Thought Disorder
14. Possession of Thought
15. Non-delusional Thoughts
16. Delusional Thoughts
17. Disorders of Perception
18. Disorder of Identity and Will
19. Attention and Concentration
20. Memory
21. Information and Intelligence
22. Risk Factors for Violence in Psychosis
23. Interview of Specific Patients and Situations
24. Clinical Risk Management

25. Cognitive State Assessment for Organic Brain Disease and Some Neurological Examinations
26. Grief, Bereavement and Complicated Grief
27. Diagnostic and Statistical Manual of Mental Disorders (DSM-5)
28. International Classification of Diseases, 10th Revision, WHO (1992)
29. Personality Disorders
30. Ego Defense Mechanisms
31. Some Pioneers of Psychoanalytical Psychiatry
32. Psychiatric Report
33. Commonly Used Rating Scales in Psychiatry
34. Commonly used Laboratory Tests in Psychiatry
35. Electrocardiogram
36. Some Clinical Syndromes
37. Some Commonly Used Terms/Conditions in Clinical Psychiatry
38. Mental Healthcare Act 2017 (India)

Appendix 1

History of Present Complaints

Predisposing factors that predisposes the individual to psychiatric disorders, e.g. genetic makeup or obstetric complications or personality

Precipitating factors that arise just before a psychiatric disorder starts, e.g. the death of a loved one or stressful life experience like breaking of a relationship or loss of job

Perpetuating factors that cause an existing psychiatric disorder to continue, e.g. social withdrawal in depression or in schizophrenia

Vegetative signs collectively refer to the disturbances of sleep, loss of appetite, weight loss, constipation and loss of sexual interest (libido) usually used in relation to depression.

Insomnia includes any combination of difficulty with falling asleep, staying asleep, intermittent wakefulness and early morning awakening. Usual causes are:
- Medical or psychiatric conditions, e.g. chronic pain, asthma, arthritic pain, heart failure, psychosis, mood disorders, depression, anxiety, panic, stress, alcoholism.
- Psychophysiological insomnia: A condition in which stress caused by the insomnia makes it even harder to fall asleep.
- Delayed sleep phase syndrome: The internal clock is constantly out of synch with the "accepted" day/night phases, e.g. patients feel best if they can sleep from 4 AM to noon.
- Hypnotic-dependent sleep disorder: Insomnia that occurs after stopping or become tolerant to certain types of sleep medications.
- Stimulant-dependent sleep disorder: Insomnia that occurs after stopping or become dependent on certain types of stimulants (caffeine, theophylline, amphetamine).

Sleep Disorders:
- *Hypersomnia:* Problems with staying awake or disorders of excessive sleepiness—common causes are idiopathic hypersomnia, narcolepsy, obstructive and central sleep apnea, restless leg syndrome.
- *Sleep rhythm problem:* Problems sticking to a regular sleep schedule—do not maintain a consistent sleep-wake schedule. This occurs when travelling between times zones (Jet lag syndrome), with shift workers on rotating schedules, particularly night time workers, paradoxical insomnia (the person actually sleeps a different amount than they think they do).
- *Parasomnia or sleep-disruptive behaviors*: Abnormal behaviors during sleep, fairly common in children, e.g. sleep terrors, sleepwalking.

APPENDIX 2

Genogram

A **genogram** is a pictorial display of a person's family tree depicting family relatedness, many basic information, current relationship as well as medical history. It goes beyond a traditional family tree. Murray Bowen had invented the concept of the genogram in the 1970s. It uses a set of predesignated symbols to convey information.

Example of a simple genogram:

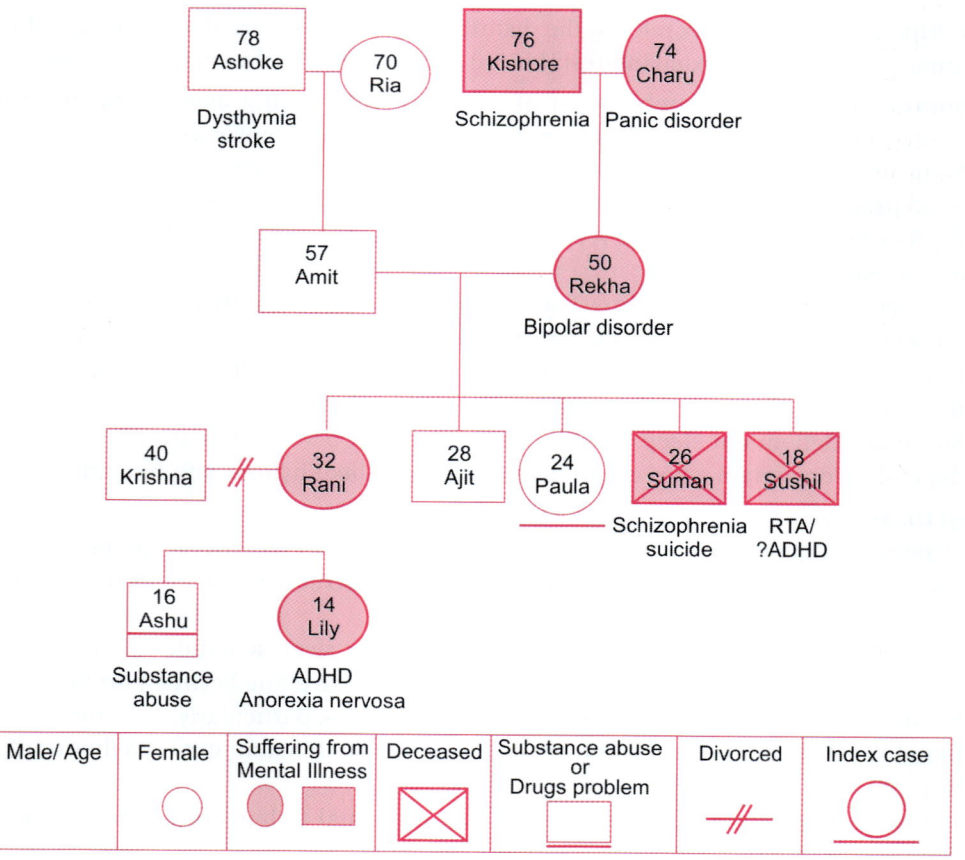

APPENDIX 3

Premenstrual Syndrome

Premenstrual Syndrome (PMS): This is a mixture of physical and emotional symptoms that some women have during the days, or sometimes weeks, leading up to their menstrual period. PMS can affect the quality of life and relationships. A more severe form is *premenstrual dysphoric disorder* (PMDD): Three groups of symptoms: *Emotional symptoms* (mood swings, depression, anxiety/irritability, feeling upset/emotional, decreased self-esteem), *physical symptoms* (headaches, backache, fluid retention and feeling bloated, muscle/joint pain, breast tenderness, and insomnia) and *behavioral symptoms* (loss of interest in sex, appetite changes or food cravings).

Premenstrual dysphoric disorder is a severe form of premenstrual syndrome. Premenstrual dysphoric disorder follows a predictable, cyclic pattern. Symptoms begin in the late luteal phase of the menstrual cycle (after ovulation) and end shortly after menstruation begins.

APPENDIX 4

Premorbid Personality

■ BEHAVIORAL CLUES OF DIFFERENT PERSONALITY TYPES

Balanced: Sound, well-regulated mind with a sense of responsibility and positive attitudes without any significant psychological defect	*Anxious (avoidant):* A pervasive pattern of social inhibition, feelings of inadequacy, extreme sensitivity to negative evaluation, and avoidance of social interaction	*Passive-aggressive:* A pervasive pattern of negative attitudes and passive usually disavowed resistance in interpersonal or occupational situations	*Paranoid:* A pervasive, long-standing suspiciousness and generalized mistrust of others
Dependent: A pervasive psychological dependence on other people	*Borderline:* Pervasive instability in moods, interpersonal relationships, self-image, and behavior	*Schizoid:* Avoid social activities and consistently shy away from interaction with others, generally loners with an inability to form personal relationships	*Schizotypal:* Odd or eccentric, and usually have few, if any, close relationships, a tendency to turn inward in social situations, respond inappropriately to social cues and hold peculiar beliefs
Cyclothymic: Frequent alternating periods of elation and depression, usually occurring spontaneously and not related to external circumstances	*Anankastic:* General psychological inflexibility, rigid conformity to rules and procedures, perfectionism, moral code, and/or excessive orderliness	*Histrionic:* Excessive emotionality and attention-seeking behavior	*Narcissistic:* Preoccupied with issues of personal adequacy, power, prestige and vanity

Personality traits: They reflect people's characteristics pattern of thoughts, feelings and behavior. According to "Five-Factor Model' of trait theory (Goldberg, 1990) these traits are an acronym as OCEAN: O for Openness; C for Consciousness; E for Extraversion; A for Agreeableness and N for Neuroticism. Big Five comprises five major traits as follows (Diener and Lucus, 2018):

Appendix 4: Premorbid Personality

Traits	Definition
Openness	The tendency to appreciate creativity, new art, values, feelings and behaviors
Consciousness	The tendency to be careful, on-time for appointments, to follow the rules, and to be hardworking
Extraversion	The tendency to be talkative, sociable, and to enjoy others, the tendency to have a dominant style
Agreeableness	The tendency to agree and go along with others rather than to assert one's own opinions and choices
Neuroticism	The tendency to frequently experience negative emotions, such as anger, worry and sadness, as well as being interpersonally sensitive

Temperament: It is the way one tends to behave or the types of emotions one tends to exhibit.

Appendix 5

Cultural Assessment in Psychiatry

Why is cultural assessment important in clinical psychiatry?
Series of anthropological, sociological and cross-cultural research has clearly demonstrated that:
- Cause, course and outcome of major psychiatric disorders are influenced by cultural factors (Kleinman, 1988; Kirmayer, 2001; Leff, 2001)
- Social and cultural factors are the major determinants of the use of healthcare services and alternative sources of help
- Culturally based attitudes and assumptions govern the perspective of both patient and clinician that influence the outcome of management
- In view of the recent global migration, most of the mental health professionals are engaged in intercultural clinical work and thus
- Cultural competence is a requisite skill of a psychiatrist to address the relevant socio-cultural perspectives in working with a culturally diverse clinical population.
- Ethnicity, ethnocultural identity, social class, cultural dimension of gender, cultural explanation and meaning of sufferings or illness, cultural codes of expression of distress, cultural value system and support, cultural belief about religion and spirituality, cultural specificity in coping mechanism and ways of intercultural assimilation are the few broad issues in cultural assessment in clinical psychiatry.

■ AIM OF CULTURAL ASSESSMENT (CHOWDHURY, 2011)
- To integrate the relevant elements of the cultural context of the patient's identity, illness experience and psychosocial context that can guide diagnosis and treatment.
- To improve the delivery of appropriate services to a culturally diverse population.
- Encourage clinical ability and precision to elicit cultural information to understand how the patients and their families cultural universe influence the course of the disorder, and to develop a treatment/care plan that empowers the patients' cultural value while allowing appropriate professional intervention.

- It is based on respect for and interest in difference (diversity) which thus helps to avoid ethnocentrism in psychiatric practice.

POINTS TO CONSIDER IN CULTURAL FORMULATION

- *Ethnocultural identity*: Individual's ethnic or cultural reference group; immigrant or ethnic minority; language, religious orientation and spirituality, any experience or feelings of discrimination; nature of social or community support available.
- *Explanatory model* about current illness: Cultural name or meaning of the symptom and behavior; any particular idioms of distress, perceived cause or mechanism, patterns of distress, type of help-seeking, expected treatment and outcome.
- *Clinician-patient relationship*: Expectations about the clinical process, cultural appropriateness of the care plan offered, working alliance.
- Assess whether there are any *communication difficulties* and cultural distance.
- Be sensitive and careful about *cultural pattern of health-seeking behaviors*, religious or social taboos.
- Assess any *acculturation effect* on present behavior. It can be assessed by focusing on religious activity, food preferences, leisure activities, attitudes to traditional patterns of behavior in the community (Goldberg and Murray, 2007).
- Any evidence of *cultural contamination* (picking up dysfunctional behavior from host culture) in symptom formation (usually found in a migrant individual).
- If needed help from an interpreter or cultural brokers may be sought for.

EXPLANATORY MODEL OF ILLNESS (EMI)

Patient's illness beliefs influence their symptom formation and degree of disability. Explanatory models are the perception of a sickness and its treatment that is employed by all those engaged in the clinical process (Kleinman et al. 1978). Weiss (1997) further developed this construct into different clinical sets of explanatory model interview catalogue (EMIC) for different cultural and clinical groups. The explanatory model is a very useful clinical tool in mental health and in medicine.

Arthur Kleinman's (1981) 8 Questions of Explanatory Framework:
1. What do you call your problem?
2. What has caused it?
3. Why do you think it started and when it did?
4. What does it do for you?
5. How severe is it?
6. What do you fear most about it?
7. What are the chief problems it has caused you?
8. What kind of treatment do you think you should receive?

Guidelines for Developing Cultural Competency (Berlin and Fowkes, 1983)
LEARN
L= Listen with sympathy and understanding to the patient's perception of the problems
E= Explain your perception of the problems
A= Acknowledge and discuss the differences and similarity
R= Recommend treatment
N= Negotiate agreement

Cultural consideration is very important for Mental State Examination (MSE), especially when it is applied in a cross-cultural context, when the clinician and patient are from different cultural backgrounds. For example, the patient's culture might have different norms for appearance, behavior, display of emotions and communication pattern. Culturally normative spiritual and religious beliefs need to be distinguished from delusions and hallucinations without understanding may seem similar though they have different roots. The cognitive assessment must also take the patient's language and educational background into account. Clinician's racial bias is another potential confounder.

The interviewer should be conscious of the most common *cultural blocks in cross-cultural communication:*
- *Ethnocentrism:* Inability to accept another culture's worldview, e.g. "my way is the best."
- *Discrimination:* Differential treatment of an individual due to minority status; actual or perceived, e.g. "we are not just equipped to serve people like that."
- *Generalization:* Reducing numerous characteristics of an individual or group to a general form that is an oversimplification.
- *Stereotyping:* Generalizing about a person while ignoring the presence of individual difference, e.g. "she is like that because she's Asian – all Asians are nonverbal."
- *Cultural Blindness:* Differences are ignored, and one proceeds as though differences did not exist, e.g. "there is no need to worry about a person's culture."
- *Cultural imposition:* It is the intrusive application of the majority group's cultural view upon individuals and families (Universal Declaration of Human Rights, 2001). The belief that everyone should conform to the majority, e.g. "we know what's best for you, if you do not like it you can go elsewhere."
- *Racism:* Race has social meaning, assigns status, limits or increase opportunities and influence interaction between patient and clinicians. The International Convention on the Elimination of All Forms of Racial Discrimination (UN, 1965) defines racism *"Any distinction, exclusion, restriction or preference based on race, colour, descent, or national or ethnic origin which has the purpose or effect of nullifying or impairing the recognition, enjoyment or exercise, on equal footing, of human rights and fundamental freedoms in the political, economic, social, cultural or any other fields of public life."* Racism may be overt or covert.

Multidisciplinary Team and Cultural Formulation
Culturally competent professionals in the multidisciplinary team (MDT) may collect and share the cultural information of the patient for devising the care plan:

- *The psychologist* may explore the worldview with a focus on cultural beliefs and practices related to health and illness,
- *The psychiatric nurse* may collect the cultural perception of current distress, past help-seeking and family involvement in the therapeutic intervention,
- *The social worker* may explore the migration history, cultural assimilation/rejection or acculturative stress (if present) and nature of social support
- *Occupational therapist* may explore the cultural notion of body image and cultural norms and values in functional (activities of daily living/taboos) assessment
- *The psychiatrist* may explore the cultural meaning and interpretation of mental symptoms, health seeking preferences in treatment negotiation.
- [DSM-5 described details of 'Cultural Formulation' under Section III (pp.749-759)]

APPENDIX 6

Physical Health Monitoring in Mental Health

The physical health of people with mental disorders and disabilities drawing a renewed clinical interest in recent years because of a series of research findings and advent of 'metabolic syndrome' as a side effect of continued antipsychotic treatment. People with mental disorders have an increased risk of poor physical health and are dying earlier than people in the general population. Eating disorders and addictions carry the highest mortality risks. Death from unnatural causes (accidents, suicide, homicide) are found higher for schizophrenia, and major depression and death from natural causes are increased in people with organic mental disorders. People with intellectual disabilities are 58 times more likely to die before age 50 (Lee and Cormac, 2012).

Poor physical health in mental patients is due to a combination of factors (Brown et al. 1999):
- Increased rates of tobacco smoking
- Increased use of alcohol and illicit substances
- Decreased levels of physical activity
- Increased rates of obesity.

Lifestyle and risk of physical health is a serious concern among patients with mental disorders. Mental health professionals should be well aware of the following issues and physical health monitoring during the treatment:
- Type 2 diabetes
- Obesity and metabolic syndrome
- Cardiovascular disease
- Drugs associated with weight gain.

Body Mass Index

It is a reliable measure in physical health monitoring. Body mass index (BMI) is calculated by dividing weight (in Kg) by height (in meters) squared. Abnormal BMI is associated with many ill health conditions like type 2 diabetes, cardiovascular disease, sleep apnea and osteoarthritis.

Management of Metabolic Syndrome

The metabolic syndrome is a cluster of risk factors for diabetes and cardiovascular disease and is a useful risk indicator for mental patients. Management is aimed at:
- Immediate therapy for all vascular risk factors
- Lifestyle measures—diet, smoking cessation, increased exercise
- Reduction of hypertension
- Management of dyslipidemia
- Rearrangement of therapeutic medication.

It is a good medical practice to follow a standard protocol for physical health monitoring for patients who are on clozapine, antipsychotic/antidepressant medications with baseline values and periodic assessments.

Royal College of Psychiatrist, London (2009) has set specific standards for psychiatrists on their role in physical health care as follows:
- Psychiatrists must be competent to undertake a physical examination and to arrange investigations.
- Psychiatrists must ensure that they understand the therapeutic and adverse effects of prescribed medications and they report suspected adverse drug reactions.

Lifestyle change is an important medical advice to our clients to enhance positive physical and mental health. Most commonly a lifestyle issue about encouraging individuals would be:
- Stop smoking
- Eat healthy food
- Maintain a healthy weight
- Drink alcohol within recommended daily limits
- Undertake regular physical activity
- Improve mental health well-being.

Appendix 7

Central Nervous System Examination

Confusion: Refers to a loss of orientation (ability to place oneself correctly in the world by time, location, and personal identity) and often memory (ability to correctly recall previous events or learn new material). Confusion interferes with the ability to make decisions.

Clouding: A state of consciousness affecting thinking, attention, and perception in which one is confused about, or not fully aware of one's immediate surroundings.

Stupor: Stupor is unresponsiveness from which a person can be aroused only by vigorous, physical stimulation. In stupor, eye movements become purposeful when the painful stimulus is applied, and wincing or pupillary constriction may occur, but the patient remains akinetic and mute.

Torpor: A lowering of consciousness short of stupor. Awareness is narrowed and restricted, and apathy, perseveration, and psychomotor retardation are observed, but the more dramatic phenomena of delirium (i.e. illusions, hallucinations, agitation, and so on) are lacking. Torpor is associated with severe infection and multi-infarct dementia.

Twilight or dreamy states: Restricted awareness is manifested as disorientation for time and place with reduced attention and short-term memory. In addition, the patient may have the sense of being in a dream.

Delirium: The patient has a reduced awareness of and responsiveness to the environment, which may be manifested as disorientation, incoherence, and memory disturbance. Delirium is often marked by hallucinations, delusions, and a dream-like state.

Coma: Coma is unresponsiveness from which a person cannot be aroused. In coma, the person's eyes remain closed.

Psychogenic coma: Psychogenic coma is suggested by normal vital and neurologic signs, resistance to opening the eyes, normal pupillary reactions, and staring (rather than wandering) eyes. Swallowing, corneal, and gag reflexes are usually intact, and electroencephalography and oculovestibular reflexes are normal.

Epileptic automatism: A state of clouding of consciousness during or immediately after a seizure, during which posture and muscle tone are maintained. The individual may perform actions without being aware of what is happening. Commonly seen in temporal lobe epilepsy.

Serotonin syndrome is potentially a life-threatening adverse drug reaction that may occur following therapeutic drug use, inadvertent interactions between drugs, overdose of particular drugs, or the recreational use of certain drugs (e.g. antidepressants, antiemetics, antimigraine drugs, over-the-counter cold remedies, recreational drugs, herbal remedies). The syndrome is the consequence of excessive stimulation of the CNS and peripheral serotonin receptors leading to excess serotonergic activity. The symptoms are of a clinical triad of abnormalities: Cognitive effects (headache, agitation, hypomania, confusion, hallucination, coma), *autonomic effects* (shivering, sweating, hyperthermia, hypertension, tachycardia, nausea, diarrhea) and *somatic effects* (myoclonus, hyper-reflexia manifested by clonus, and tremor).

International Classification of Epilepsy

Generalized seizures: Primary generalized seizures appear to have a bilateral onset in the cerebral cortex. If a seizure begins locally and then evolves into a generalized seizure, it is called a secondary generalized seizure	*Absence seizures (petit mal)*: Occur without warning and consist of a sudden interruption of consciousness, common in childhood and adolescence
	Tonic-clonic seizures (grand mal): Prodrome and aura → loss of consciousness → tonic phase → incontinence urine or feces, dilated pupil unreactive to light—this phase lasts for 10-60 seconds → clinic phase with autonomic signs—last from few seconds to few minutes → postictal phase—unresponsive for a variable period of time → period of drowsiness and disorientation
	Tonic or clonic seizures
	Atonic seizures: Brief loss of muscle tone which may be generalized (causing fall) or may be localized. Known as 'drop attack'.
	Myoclonic seizures: A sudden, brief, shock-like involuntary muscle contraction may produce a generalized or focal jerk
Partial seizures (focal or local seizures): No alteration of consciousness unless it evolves into secondary generalized seizures	*Simple partial seizures*: Simple motor seizures/simple sensory seizures/other simple partial seizures
	Complex partial seizures: Temporal lobe seizures/Frontal lobe seizures
	Partial seizures evolving to secondary generalized seizures
C. *Unclassified seizures*	

Different Stages of a Seizure Episode

- *Prodrome:* A vague sense that a seizure is imminent and may last for hours or days.
- *Aura:* The subjective sensation that precedes and mark the onset of the seizure. May point to the localization of the site in the brain.
- *Ictus:* The seizure
- *Postictal phase*: Abnormal state after the ictus until a full recovery.

Appendix 8

General Appearance and Behavior

- *General appearance*: Following features may suggest psychiatric importance:
  - General self-neglect → chronic schizophrenia, dementia, alcohol/drug addiction.
  - Bright/colorful clothing → mania
  - Stooped, hunched, leaning forward → depression
  - Sitting on the edge of the seat, gripping the arms of the chair, restless and fidgety → anxiety/ADHD.
- *Facial expressions:* A sad face with downturned corners of the mouth, flattened expressions and vertical furrowing of the brows suggests depression/horizontal furrowing of the brow with wide eyes, sweating and dilated pupils suggests anxiety/an expressionless, mask-like face suggests the parkinsonian syndrome/Graves' disease is characterized by exophthalmos.
- *Movements:* Some movements are characteristics of the psychiatric disorder as in: Depressive affective disorder (slow, ponderous movements/in extreme cases there may be immobility and mutism (stupor), mania (movements are rapid and pressured/overactivity and restlessness), anxiety (restless/tremulous movements) and Parkinsonism (difficulty in initiating movement or slow, stiff movements), fidgety and uncomfortable in seating (ADHD).
- *Waxy flexibility:* Characterized by a patient's movements having the feeling of a plastic resistance, as if the person were made of wax. This occurs in catatonic schizophrenia.
- *Ambitendency:* A tendency to act in opposite ways or directions, i.e. the presence of opposing behavioral drives.
- *Mannerisms:* Repeated involuntary movements that appear to be goal-directed.
- *Grimaces:* A distorted facial expression of disgust, pain or displeasure.
- *Negativism:* Patient resists attempts to move him and does opposite to what is asked. It is usually a sign of catatonia.
- *Eye contact:* Eye contact is a form of nonverbal communication that largely influences the social behavior. The customs and significance of eye contact vary widely between cultures and religion. Eye contact may be reduced in depression, unsettling in autistic disorder or social anxiety, may appear staring in patients suffering from Parkinsonian drug side effects.

- *Episodes of aggression/crying*: Initially or during the interview
- *Distraction*: From the clinical consultation (marked in ADHD)
- *Rapport:* This is a measure of the quality of the interaction between the patient and the examiner. Try to describe the actual characteristics of the interaction and how it changes throughout the interview.

Appendix 9

Language Evaluation

Aphasia: Acquired impairments of the lexical or syntactical aspect of language (comprehension or expression) produced by brain dysfunction, usually described as fluent and non-fluent.

Fluent aphasia (Receptive aphasia): Reflect dysfunction in the left temporal and parietal area and is characterized by the production of many well-articulated phrases with normal prosody but yields little informational content. Examples are Wernicke's aphasia, anomic aphasia, conduction aphasia, transcortical sensory aphasia.

Wernicke's aphasia: Fluent, effortless, well-articulated speech. Severe disturbances in comprehension, repetition, impaired naming—paraphasic—hence sometimes considered psychotic. Prognosis for language recovery is poor.

Anomic aphasia: Occurs in—Alzheimer's disease, head injury, metabolic encephalopathy. Localization significance is limited. Prognosis for language recovery depends on the severity of the initial defect. Main defect—word finding difficulty and inability to name objects on confrontation.

Conduction aphasia: A disproportionate deficit in repetition. Good comprehension and reading, but naming is mildly disturbed.

Semantic aphasia: Complete word substitution (pen for the car)

Phonemic aphasia: Substitution of a syllable (lar for car)

Jargon aphasia: Heavily paraphasic but fluent speech.

Non-fluent aphasia (Expressive aphasia): Reflects lesions anterior left hemisphere, characterized by slow and poor verbal output, difficulty with spontaneous speech, omissions of grammatical connecting words and poor prosody. Examples are Broca's aphasia, global aphasia, transcortical motor aphasia.

Broca's aphasia: Non-fluent dysarthric dysprosodic effortful speech. Repetition, reading speech and spontaneous speech severely impaired. Auditory and reading comprehension remains intact. Likely to have an anterior left hemispheric lesion.

Global aphasia: Most common and severe form. Large lesions that damage most of the perisylvian area including frontal and parietotemporal language areas.

Pure aphasias: Selective impairments in reading, writing, or the recognition of words. For example, a person is able to read but not write, or is able to write but not read. Examples are Pure alexia, agraphia, pure word deafness.

Pure alexia: Severe reading problems while other language-related skills such as naming, oral repetition, auditory comprehension or writing are typically intact.

Agraphia (Dysgraphia): Is a deficiency in the ability to write, regardless of the ability to read, not due to intellectual impairment.

Pure word deafness: Inability to comprehend the meaning of speech, but (in most cases) still able to hear, speak, read, and write. It is caused by bilateral damage to the posterior superior temporal lobes or disruption of connections between these areas.

Aprosodias: Nonverbal aspects of speech, the melody, pauses, timing, stress, accent and intonation is disturbed. Right prefrontal damage → expressive aprosodias and right temporal and insular damage → receptive aprosodias.

Clinicopathological Pattern in Aphasias

Aphasia type	Speech	Repetition	Comprehension	Naming	Area of lesion
Broca's	Nonfluent	X	√	X	Left posterior-inferior frontal
Wernicke's	Fluent	X	X	X- often	Left posterior-superior temporal
Conduction	Fluent	X	X	X- often	Left supramarginal gyrus or left auditory cortex
Global	Nonfluent	X	X	X	Left frontal parietal temporal
Transcortical motor	Nonfluent	√	X	X	Left frontal, anterior or superior to Broca's area
Transcortical sensory	Fluent	√	X	X	Left temporoparietal areas surrounding Wernicke's area
Anomic	Fluent	√	√	X	Left temporoparietal or frontal
Subcortical	Fluent + articulatory defect	√/ X	X	√/ X	Caudate; thalamus

X = Impaired; √ = Intact

Appendix 10

Voice and Speech

Aphonia: Speaks but fails to produce any volume of sound or merely whispers. Found in disorders of the larynx and vocal cord. If, despite this, the patient is able to cough normally, the origin is probably hysterical.

Dysphonia: Difficulty or pain in speaking.

Dysarthria: Volume of sound and content is normal, but the articulation and enunciation of individual words and phrases are distorted. Found in disorders of control of muscles producing speech—upper or lower motor neuron lesions.

Dysphasia: Failure to put properly constructed words or phrases for expression. The lesion is in the dominant cerebral hemisphere. Dysphasic state also includes disturbances of writing (dysgraphia) and failure to comprehend the spoken word (receptive dysphasia) or the written word (dyslexia).

Slow speech: May be a feature of retardation. Usually associated with a lack of spontaneous and reduced speed of reply.

Fast speech: Often results from 'normal' anxiety but may indicate mania or schizophrenia.

Pressure of speech: Rapid speech that is increased in amount and difficult to interrupt.

Push of speech: Rapid speech that is increased in amount but can be interrupted.

Volubility (logorrhea): Copious, coherent and logical speech.

Poverty of speech: Restriction in the amount of speech, replies may be monosyllabic.

Nonspontaneous speech: Verbal responses given only when asked or spoken to directly, no self-initiation of speech.

Poverty of content of speech: Speech is adequate in amount but covers little information because of vagueness, emptiness or stereotyped phrases.

Dysprosody: Loss of normal speech melody (called prosody)

Stuttering (Stammering): Frequent repetition or prolongation of a sound or syllabi leading to markedly impaired speech fluency.

Muttering: A low continuous indistinct sound; often accompanied by movement of the lips without the production of articulate speech.

Slurring speech: Or difficulty articulating words, commonly associated with drunkenness. Other causes are drug intoxication, hypoglycemic attacks, brain pathologies like stroke or TIA and physical disorders of the face or oral region that interfere with speech. Slurred speech is not the same as poorly articulated speech or overly rapid speech.

Bradylalia: Abnormally slow speech.

Paraphasia: Abnormal speech in which one word is substituted for another two types: (1) *Semantic paraphasia*: Problem in the selection of right word thus substituted a word (words) for the correct one; (2) *Phonemic paraphasia*: Does errors by adding or omitting phonemes or mis-sequencing the order of the phonemes in a word (treen for train).

Allusory speech: Vague, imprecise and hard to comprehend speech because too few details are provided.

Rhyming: Using words that sound alike, as used in poetry—not italics

Punning: A play on words, sometimes on different senses of the same word and sometimes on the similar sense or sound of different words.

Clang association: A thought disorder wherein words are chosen or repeated based on similar sounds, instead of semantic meaning.

Cryptolalia: A private language, which is spoken aloud.

Telegraphic speech: Conjunctions and articles are missed out in a sentence but the meaning is retained, and few words are used.

Mutism: The inability or unwillingness to speak. Mutism are of two types. Akinetic mutism—a state in which a person is unspeaking (mute) and unmoving (akinetic). A person with akinetic mutism has sleep-waking cycles but, when apparently awake, with eyes open, lies mute, immobile and unresponsive. Akinetic mutism is often due to damage to the frontal lobes of the brain. Selective mutism is a childhood disorder in which a child does not speak in some social situations although he or she is able to talk normally at other times.

Appendix 11

Catatonia

■ CATATONIA

Catatonia is a state of motor immobility and behavioral abnormality, commonly manifested by stupor and was first described by Karl Ludwig Kahlbaum (28.12.1828-15.4.1899), a German psychiatrist in 1874 in his monograph 'Die Katatonie oder das Spannungsirresein' (Catatonia or Tension Insanity). Catatonia is a neuropsychiatric syndrome that can occur due to medical or psychiatric disorder. Rajagopal (2007) provided a very comprehensive review of Catatonia. The three main clinical types are Catatonic Stupor, Catatonic Excitement and Malignant Catatonia. The main symptoms of catatonia (adopted from Rajagopal, 2007) are as follows:

Clinical features	Description
Stupor	It is a motionless motor immobility with nonreactivity to external stimuli, often accompanied by mutism and rigidity
Posturing	Patient maintains the same posture for long periods
Waxy flexibility (cereal flexinilitas)	Patient maintains highly uncomfortable postures for long periods of time
Negativism	Patient resists the attempt to move parts of their body and the resistance offered is equal to the strength applied
Automatic obedience	Patient demonstrates exaggerated cooperation, automatically obeying every instruction of the clinician
Ambitendency	Patient alternates between resistance to and cooperation with the clinician's instruction (e.g. when asked to shake hands, the patient repeatedly extends and withdraws hands)
Forced grasping	The patient forcibly and repeatedly grasps the clinician's hand when offered
Obstruction	The patient stops suddenly in the course of a movement and is generally unable to offer any reason. This appears to be the motor counterpart of thought block
Echopraxia	The patient imitates the action of the interviewer
Aversion	The patient turns away from the examiner when addressed
Mannerisms	Repetitive goal-directed movements (e.g. saluting)

Contd...

Contd...

Clinical features	Description
Stereotypies	Repetitive, non-goal directed regular movements (e.g. rocking)
Motor perseveration	The patient persists with a particular movement that has lost its initial relevance
Excitement	Patient displays excessive, purposeless motor activity that is not influenced by external stimuli
Speech abnormalities	Three main speech abnormalities: *Echolalia*: repetition of the examiner's words; *Logorrhoea*: incessant, incoherent and monotonous speech; *Verbigeration*: a form of verbal perseveration in which the patient repeats certain syllables (*logoclonia*), words (*palilalia*) or phrases or sentences
Malignant catatonia	Is an acute onset of excitement with fever, autonomic instability, delirium and may be fatal

For diagnosis of Catatonic Schizophrenia in ICD 10 (category F20.2) requires that the patient prominently exhibits at least one of the following catatonic features, for at least 2 weeks: stupor, excitement, posturing, negativism, rigidity, waxy flexibility and command automatism (automatic obedience). DSM IV categorizes catatonia as a subtype of schizophrenia (295.20), a specifier for affective disorders, as well as a catatonic disorder secondary to a general medical condition (293.89), which is also referred to as "secondary catatonia." The diagnosis of 'schizophrenia, catatonic type' is made if the clinical picture is dominated by at least two of the following: Motor immobility, excessive motor activity, extreme negativism, peculiarities of voluntary movements, and echolalia/echopraxia. The catatonic subtype, as also the other subtypes of schizophrenia has been eliminated in DSM-5. Instead, a catatonic specifier has been added and may be used with depressive, bipolar, and psychotic disorders. This change recognizes that catatonia occurs across several categories of disorders, without necessarily indicating psychosis. In addition, there are two new catatonic disorders: Catatonic disorder due to another medical condition and other specified catatonic disorder, has been added.

Catatonia carries a high health risk: Profound negativism, immobility, and refusal to take in fluids predisposes patients to malnutrition, dehydration, rhabdomyolysis, aspiration pneumonia, obstructive nephropathy, azotemia, deep vein thrombosis (DVT), and pulmonary embolism; Immobility for prolonged period may increase the risk of deep-vein thrombosis; increased risk of death due to pulmonary embolism in patients with persistent catatonia has been reported (McCall et al. 1995) and during catatonic excitement, the patient may pose a significant risk of harm to self and others.

APPENDIX 12

Mood and Affect

Some other mood types: Aggressive, ambitious, ashamed, amused, bitter, bleak, boisterous, bright, brooding, calm/peaceful, careless, cheerful, confident, confrontational, cynical/sarcastic, dysphoric (an unpleasant mood, such as sadness, anxiety, or irritability), delicate, dramatic, energetic, enigmatic, exciting, elegant, fierce, fractured, fun, gentle, gleeful, gloomy, happy, harsh, humorous, light, lively, malevolent, outraged, paranoid, playful, precious, provocative, raucous, rebellious, reckless, relaxed, reserved, restrained, romantic, rowdy, sentimental, sexy, silly, somber, soothing, spiritual, spooky, stylish, theatrical, volatile, warm, whimsical, witty.

■ DEFINITIONS OF DISTURBANCES OF AFFECT

Blunted: A severe reduction in the intensity of emotional expression.

Fixed: Display of only one particular emotion and absence of range and mobility of affect.

Flat: Near-absence of affective expression—emotionally dull, monotonous, and lacking in resonance?

Inappropriate: Emotional expression and thought content do not coincide.

Incongruous: Affect not in keeping with the topic being discussed.

Labile: Repeated, rapid and abrupt variability in affective expression occurs.

Restricted or constricted: Mild to moderate reduction in emotional expression.

Affective incontinence: Complete loss of control and there is an expression of emotion in the absence of any adequate cause, indicative of organic brain pathology.

Apathy: A dulled emotional tone associated with detachment or indifference (also known as anergia), may be observed in patients with pre-schizophrenic, schizophrenic, depressive, and organic brain disorders.

Histrionic affect: The blatant but rather shallow expression of emotion- often encountered in people with histrionic, narcissistic, or borderline personality disorder.

la belle indifférence (literally, 'beautiful indifference'): A naive, inappropriate lack of emotion or concern for the perceptions by others of one's disability, usually seen in persons with conversion disorder.

Catastrophic reaction: Are emotional outbursts or explosions accompanied by tears or anger or by physical acting-out behavior, which seem inappropriate or out of proportion to the situation, usually occur in organically impaired individuals, when they cannot perform simple tasks.

Bipolar affective disorder (www.rcpsych.ac.uk/PDF/Bipolar%20BDF.pdf): Bipolar disorder used to be called 'manic depression'. Someone with bipolar disorder will have severe mood swings. These usually last several weeks or months and are far beyond the usual normal range.

Types of Mood
- *Low or depressive*: Feelings of intense depression and despair
- *High or manic*: Feelings of extreme happiness and elation
- *Mixed:* Mix of the above two in any combination, e.g. depressed mood with the restlessness and overactivity of a manic episode.

Clinical Types
- *Bipolar I:* There has been at least one high or manic episode, which has lasted for longer than one week. Some people with Bipolar I will have only manic episodes, although most will also have periods of depression. Untreated, manic episodes generally last 3 to 6 months. Depressive episodes last rather longer—6 to 12 months without treatment.
- *Bipolar II:* There has been more than one episode of severe depression, but only mild manic episodes—these are called 'hypomania'.

Rapid Cycling
More than four mood swings happen in a 12-month period. This affects around 1 in 10 people with bipolar disorder and can happen with both types I and II.

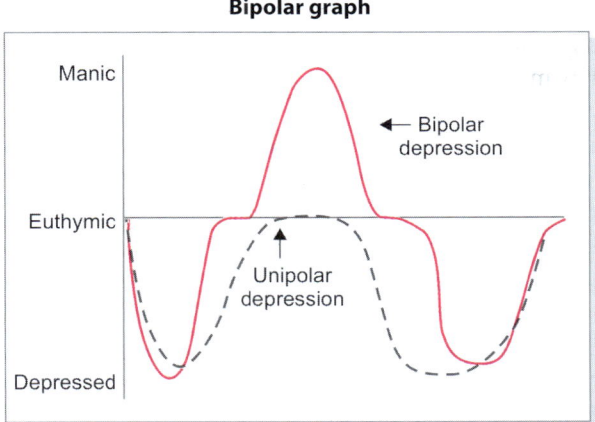

Bipolar graph

(Source: http://sharingbipolar.com/info/living-and-coping-with-bipolar-disorder/)

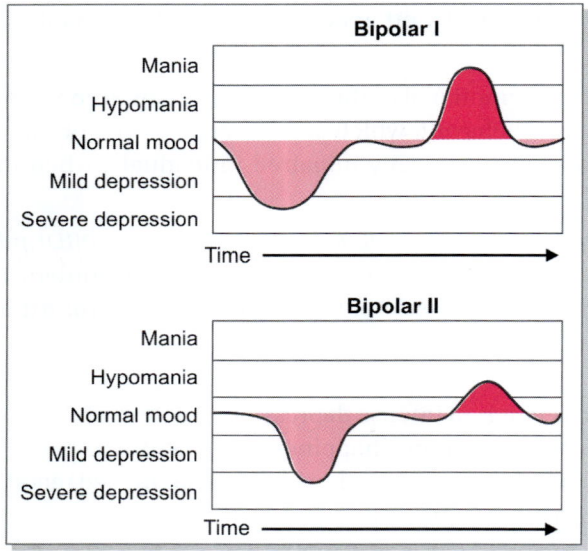

(Source: http://www.leeharrisfuhrwerk.com/2010_02_21_archive.html)

■ MOOD SWINGS

They are characterized by a drastic change in emotion from one side of the spectrum to the other. Mood swings are commonly associated with affective disorders (bipolar disorder and depression). Also seen in ADHD, borderline personality disorder (BPD), alcohol drinking, premenstrual syndrome, and menopause. Mood swings (switching) during antidepressant therapy is a serious concern in the treatment of bipolar depression.

Differential Diagnosis of Mood Swings

- *Mood swings in borderline personality disorder:* BPD is one of the Cluster B personality disorders, which are marked by dramatic, emotional or erratic behavior. Bipolar affective disorder (BAD) is a brain disorder, while BPD is an emotional disorder. Both disorders are characterized by mood swings, but the length and intensity of these mood swings are different.
    - Mood swings in BAD is due to change in neurotransmitters in the brain and seem to occur out of nowhere but in BPD mood dysregulation is a reaction to perceived environmental stress—happens in reaction to an external trigger, which are often related to perceived rejection or feelings of abandonment by a significant one (rejection sensitive dysphoria).
    - Persons with BAD typically endures the same mood for days or weeks at a time, but a person with BPD may experience intense bouts of anger, depression, and anxiety that may last only hours, or at most a day (emotional roller coaster).
    - Bipolar mood shifts are distinguished by manic episodes of elation, but BPD mood shifts rarely involve feelings of elation.

- Mood swings in BPD patients typically have a destructive character (as they have very low self-esteem and self-worth), which is manifested in frequent impulsive self-harming behavior like cutting or burning or drug overdosing, etc.
- *Mood swings in adult ADHD*: ADHD often exist with BAD comorbidity. Approximately 20% of the adults with BAD have ADHD (Perugi et al. 2013).
  - Course and phenomenology are different in BAD and ADHD: ADHD starts before age 7, and the symptoms like inattention/distractibility and/or high impulsivity/physical restlessness are the main features. BAD usually starts after puberty.
  - Triggered mood instability in ADHD by life events. BAD mood shifts are not usually connected with life events.
  - There is a mood congruency in ADHD—happy events result in a happy and excited mood and unhappy events lead to dysphoric mood.
  - Rapid mood shifting: As the mood swings are event dependent, so the ADHD mood swings are rapid in onset as well as rapid in vanishing. ADHD patients usually described this as "crashes" or "snaps". In BAD, the mood swings are untriggered and take hours or days to move from one state to another.
  - Both disorders run in families, but people with BAD usually have a family history of BAD while individuals with ADHD have a family tree with multiple cases of ADHD.
- *Premenstrual, pregnancy and menopausal mood swings:*
  - The symptoms of premenstrual syndrome (PMS) usually happen at the same time of menstrual cycle each month. This can be up to two weeks before the periods start and disappear until the next cycle starts again. Among the host of psychological and behavioral symptoms, mood swing is one.
  - Mood changes during pregnancy can be caused by physical stresses, changes in metabolism and hormones—estrogen and progesterone. Hormonal changes affect the neurotransmitters in the brain that regulate mood. Mood swings are mostly experienced during the first trimester and then again in the third trimester.
  - Mood swings are one of the symptoms of menopause. Mood swings, along with hot flushes and night sweats, are triggered by the drop in the levels of the hormones estrogen and progesterone.
- *Other disorders:* Mood swings may be found in epilepsy, autism, Parkinson's disease, Alzheimer disease, multiple sclerosis and Huntington's disease.

Anhedonia: Is an inability to experience pleasurable emotions from normally pleasurable life events such as eating, exercise, social interaction or sexual activities. This is considered as one of the negative symptoms of schizophrenia where patients describe themselves as feeling emotionally empty. It is also seen in mood disorders, schizoaffective disorders and schizoid personality disorder.

Dysthymia: Is a type of low-grade chronic depression but with less severity than major depressive disorder which lasts for several years.

Cyclothymia: Persistent instability of mood involving numerous periods of depression and mild elation but not severe or prolonged enough for a diagnosis of bipolar affective disorder or recurrent depressive disorder.

Alexithymia: Alexithymia literally means "lacking words for feelings". It is the inability to identify and express or describe one's feelings. People with alexithymia typically display a lack of imaginative thought, have difficulty distinguishing between emotions and bodily sensations, and engage in logical externally oriented thought. Usually found in somatoform disorders.

Solastalgia (Albrecht et al. 2007): is the emotional distress produced by environmental change impacting on people which are directly connected to their home environment. Nostalgia—the melancholia or homesickness experienced by individuals when separated from a loved home.

Acathexis: Lack of feeling associated with an inordinarily emotionally charged subject (in cathexis the feeling is connected).

Decathexis: Detaching emotions from thoughts, ideas or persons.

Normal stages of grief: Shock and numbness → denial → anxious searching (e.g. pseudo hallucination of bereavement) → depression and acceptance.

Complicated grief: Phobic avoidance of any place, persons or things related to the deceased/extreme guilt and anger about the deceased and the death/physical illness/recurrent nightmares about the deceased.

Appendix 13

Formal Thought Disorder

- *Loosening of association (LOA):* A disturbance of thinking in which the association of ideas and thought patterns becomes so vague, fragmented, diffuse, and unfocused as to lack any logical sequences or relationship to any preceding concepts or themes. Related terms are derailment, disjointed speech, loss of goal, flight of ideas, racing thoughts (coherent thoughts that are moving rapidly). LOA is a hallmark feature of schizophrenia.
- *Paragrammatism:* Ungrammatical word sequences.
- *Pressured speech:* Speech produced at an abnormally high rate, rapid speech that is difficult to interrupt, usually loud and intense. Characteristic for mania.
- *Racing thoughts:* A subjective sense of one's thoughts going so fast that they're hard to keep track of, may or may not be associated with pressured speech. Seen in obsession, anxiety, substance-abusing patients undergoing detoxification.
- *Echolalia:* Repetitions of a sentence just uttered by the examiner.
- *Palilalia:* Repetitions of only the last uttered word or phrase said by the examiner.
- *Poverty of speech or thought:* Reduced conversational output, very little spontaneous speech.
- *Verbigeration*: The disappearance of understandable speech, replaced by strings of incoherent utterances.
- *Word salad:* An extreme version of LOA in which changes in topic are so extreme and the associations so loose that the resulting speech is completely incoherent. Related terms: Incoherence, neologisms, Clang associations.
- *Stereotypy:* Constant repetition of a phrase (or behavior) in many different settings, irrespective of context.
- *Concrete thinking:* Literal interpretation and understanding of metaphorical expressions.
- *Illogical thinking:* A breakdown in reasoning.
- *Over-inclusive thinking:* Tendency to include items which are only remotely relevant into the stream of thoughts, i.e. inability to preserve conceptual boundaries.
- *Fusion:* Various thoughts are fused together, leading to a loss of goal direction.
- *Metonyms:* Are word approximations, e.g. paper skate for pen, eyes—for sight.
- *Condensation*: A single symbol or word is associated with the emotional content of several, not necessarily related, ideas, feelings, memories, or impulses, especially as expressed in dreams.

Appendix 14

Possession of Thought

Thought control: Other people or forces controlling or directing one's thought.

Thought insertion: Other person or forces are implanting thoughts in a person's mind.

Thought withdrawal: Other person or forces are removing thoughts from a person's mind, or thoughts have been stolen from one's mind. This is also known as thought alienation.

Thought broadcasting: One's own thoughts experienced as being transmitted to another person or agency.

Thought echo: Hearing one's own thought being spoken aloud.

Thought diffusion: Belief that as he/she is thinking, everyone else is thinking in unison with him/her (everyone else is participating in his/her thoughts).

Magical thinking: An irrational belief that thoughts can change external events without intervening actions.

Referential thinking: Perceptions of other people's actions or speech are directed to or are in reference to the self.

Thought alienation: The patient feels that his thoughts are under control of an outside agency.

APPENDIX 15

Non-delusional Thoughts

Suicidal thought or intent or self-harm thought: "Do you have any thoughts of wanting to harm or kill yourself?" or *Homicidal ideation or intent* ("Do you have any thoughts of wanting to hurt anyone?") should be inquired in detail. Please note that if there is any indication of current suicidal or homicidal ideation the person must have a thorough risk assessment and management.

Homicidal ideation or thoughts: Spans from vague ideas of revenge to detailed plans without any act (Thienhaus and Piasecki, 1998) should always be taken seriously. Homicidal thoughts in response to command hallucination is an important component of risk assessment in psychotic patients. An apprehension of hurting or harming others is seen as an obsessive rumination as well.

Worthlessness and hopelessness: Worthlessness is a pattern of subjective thinking where the individual thinks that he/she is without any worth; of no use, importance, or value and is good-for-nothing. *Hopelessness* causes the individual to believe that they are trapped in misery with no expectation of things ever getting better. It is a feeling that the present conditions will never improve, that there is no solution to a problem, and, for many, a feeling that dying by suicide would be better than living ("There are no solutions to my problems" or "I just want to give up"). Both are signs of depressive thinking. Beck (1988) developed a scale for hopelessness (20 item self-report inventory). Beck's 'Four Ds' in depression are Feelings of Defeated, Defective, Deserted, and Deprived.

Guilt/sin: Guilt is a normal emotion that is expressed as self-reproach and remorse for one's behavior, as if one violated a moral principle (Klass, 1987). Guilt, whether imagined or real, is an important thought content in major depressive disorder, post-traumatic stress disorder (PTSD) and anxiety (pathological guilt). Guilt is an important factor in perpetuating obsessive-compulsive symptoms (Shapiro and Stewart, 2011). The feeling of guilt has a number of negative psychological impacts. It erodes self-esteem and confidence, creates self-doubt and adds negative emotions such as feelings of shame, blame and worthlessness. Guilt may be of different types such as introspective guilt (bringing awareness of guilt-laden act or thoughts), perceived guilt (false sense of guilt), retrospective guilt (discovering some past issues) and religious guilt (concept of sin and punishment by God) and pathological guilt (out of proportion to the real or imagined event or act).

Free-floating anxiety: A sense of dread and/or impending doom or preoccupation with a health-related or situational factor in anxiety disorder.

Obsession: Repetitive preoccupation with a *thought,* acknowledged by the patient to be irrational and associated with anxiety. Main five types of obsession:
1. Ruminations—single or series of thoughts around a theme
2. Imagery—distressing images often of erotic nature involving relatives
3. Ideas—distressing ideas
4. Memories—distressing
5. Impulses—a feeling to hurt people or set fire

The most common obsessions are thinking or feeling objects are dirty or contaminated/worrying about health and hygiene/fear about safety and security, e.g. doors left unlocked or appliances left switched on/preoccupation with order and symmetry/religious or anti-religious thoughts/disturbing thoughts about aggression or sex/the urge to hoard useless things/superstitions; excessive attention to something considered lucky or unlucky.

Compulsion: Repetitive acts based on obsession. The most common compulsions are: Cleaning and washing, either self (hand washing), or surroundings/excessive double-checking of things (locks, appliances, switches)/repeatedly checking in on loved ones to make sure they are safe/counting, tapping, repeating certain words, or doing other senseless things to reduce anxiety/ordering things for symmetry or exactness/mental compulsions (repeating certain phrases or prayers in one's mind)/hoarding or collecting things that are useless.

Most people with obsessive-compulsive disorder fall into one of the following categories:
- *Washers*: Afraid of contamination, usually have cleaning or handwashing compulsions.
- *Checkers*: Repeatedly check things (oven turned off, door locked, etc.) that they associate with harm or danger.
- *Doubters and sinners*: Afraid that if everything is not perfect or done just right, something terrible will happen or they will be punished.
- *Counters and arrangers*: Obsessed with order and symmetry may have superstitions about certain numbers, colors, or arrangements.
- *Hoarders*: Fear that something bad will happen if they throw anything away, compulsively hoard things that they do not need or use.

Persons with traits of obsessionality may have anankastic personality. Often they overlap.

Phobia: Persistent and irrational fear of delineated aspects of nonhuman object or environment. Common three types:
1. *Simple phobia*: Fear of animals, heights, bridges, etc.
2. *Social phobia*: Fear of social situations where he/she may do a wrong thing, being looked at or asked to speak
3. *Agoraphobia*: Fear of open spaces or crowds

Other patterns of thinking: Following five types may be seen as a pattern of thinking, strongly held, not always illogical and culturally inappropriate, usually occur singly and unassociated with other psychopathology—carefully distinguish whether such thoughts have reached delusional intensity.
1. *Overvalued ideas:* Unreasonable, sustained false beliefs or ideas maintained less firmly than a delusion (i.e. the person is able to acknowledge the possibility that the belief may not be true). The belief is not one that is ordinarily accepted by other members of the person's culture or subculture. Clinical difficulties often arise to separate it from delusion.
2. *Grandiosity:* Beliefs that one's ideas, capacities or actions are generally superior to those of others.
3. *Mystical experience:* Feels that the mystery of the universe has been suddenly revealed to him, may be associated with superior power and regarded as very valuable and auspicious.
4. *Suspiciousness:* A cautious attitude based on possible malevolent intuitions of others. Simple suspiciousness is not paranoia, not if it is based on past experience or expectations learned from the experience of others.
5. *Paranoia:* Level of suspiciousness altering thinking and behavior in nonadaptive ways. It is a mistrust that is either highly exaggerated or not warranted at all.

Idea is a mental impression or conception that potentially or actually exists in the mind as a product of mental activity. Usual five types are:
1. *Autochthonous idea*: A persistent idea originating within the mind but seeming to have come from an outside source and often, therefore, felt to be of malevolent origin.
2. *Dominant idea*: One that controls or colors every action and thought.
3. *Fixed idea*: A persistent morbid impression or belief that cannot be changed by reason.
4. *Overvalued idea*: A false or exaggerated belief sustained beyond reason or logic but with less rigidity than a delusion, also often being less patently unbelievable.
5. *Idea of reference*: The incorrect idea that the words and actions of others refer to oneself or the projection of the causes of one's own imaginary difficulties upon someone else.

Overvalued idea: First described by German neurologist Carl Wernicke (1848–1905), who refers to a solitary, abnormal belief that is neither delusional nor obsessional in nature, but which is preoccupying to the extent of dominating the sufferer's life (McKenna, 1984). The relationship between delusions and overvalued ideas is complex and uncertain and thus has clinical as well as conceptual implications. Richard and Richard (2010) provided the following distinction between delusion and overvalued ideas:
- Deluded individuals are less likely to identify what might modify their belief, less preoccupied, and less concerned about others' reactions than those with overvalued ideas.
- Delusions are less plausible and their onset less likely to appear reasonable.
- Delusions are more likely to have an abrupt onset and overvalued ideas a gradual onset.
- Conviction and insight were similar in both the groups.
- Belief conviction and insight may be an inadequate basis for separating delusions from overvalued ideas. Abrupt onset, implausible content, and relative indifference to the opinions of others may be better distinguishing features.

Veale (2002) provided the following features for overvalued ideas:
- Is held strongly, with less than delusional intensity but could progress to delusion.
- Usually preoccupies the individual's thinking process.
- Is ego-syntonic, compared to most obsessions.
- Often develops in an abnormal personality.
- Is usually comprehensible with knowledge of the individual's past experience and personality.
- The content is usually regarded as abnormal compared to the general population (but not bizarre as some delusions).
- Causes disturbed functioning or distress to the patient and others.
- Is associated with a high degree of affect (e.g. anxiety or anger when there is a threat to the loss of their goal or object of the belief).
- Compared to many delusions, is more likely to lead to repeated action which is considered as justified.
- Patients may not seek help from mental health services but may be brought to the attention of the services by a concerned relative or another agency.
- Have some similarities to passionate religious or political convictions where the individual usually remains functional.

Hypochondriasis: Is excessive fear and anxiety of having a serious disease. These fears are not relieved when a medical examination finds no evidence of disease. They are often able to acknowledge that their fears are unrealistic, but this intellectual realization is not enough to reduce their anxiety. Most people occasionally fear they have an illness, but people with hypochondriasis are constantly preoccupied with their fear. This fear is severe and persistent and interferes with work as well as relationships and frequently leads to multiple health consultations. *Persistent belief* in specific ill health and *persistent refusal* of advice and reassurance is the hallmark of hypochondriasis.

Usually, hypochondriasis is the manifestation of an overvalued idea, with obsessive rumination and is frequently associated with depressive illness or chronic anxiety.

Munchausen syndrome: It is a factitious disorder characterized by the deliberate fabrication of physical/mental symptoms for no apparent reason, other than to assume a patient role. They also show up frequently in the emergency department and demands treatment.

Dysmorphophobia: The affected person is excessively concerned about and preoccupied with a perceived defect in his or her physical features (body image). Now it is known as body dysmorphic disorder (BDD). In cases where a minor defect truly exists, the individual with BDD exhibits an inordinate amount of anguish. BDD is often encountered in dermatologic and cosmetic surgery settings.

Eating disorders: Eating disorders are characterized by an abnormal attitude and beliefs towards food that causes someone to change their eating habits and behavior. They may focus excessively on their weight and shape, leading them to make unhealthy choices about food with damaging results to their health. Eating disorders include a range of conditions

that can affect someone physically, psychologically and socially. The most common eating disorders are:
- *Anorexia nervosa*: When someone tries to keep their weight as low as possible, for example, by starving themselves or exercising excessively. It is a form of *weight phobia* (fear of increasing body weight) with abnormal self-image. Important features are body weight at least 15% below that expected level; self-induced weight loss, delayed or arrested puberty and amenorrhea.
- *Bulimia nervosa*: Gross preoccupation with food; when someone tries to control his or her weight by binge eating and then deliberately being sick or using laxatives. There is marked dissatisfaction with the body.
- *Binge eating*: When someone feels compelled to overeat.
- *Compulsive overeating*: Characterized as an "addiction" to food, using food and eating as a way to hide from their emotions, to fill a void they feel inside, and to cope with daily stresses and problems in their lives.

Please note that eating disorders may sometime reach to a psychotic proportion.

APPENDIX 16

Delusional Thoughts

■ DIFFERENT TYPES OF DELUSIONS

- **Paranoid delusions:** Most common single delusion, affecting about 60% of patients.
  - *Persecutory delusion:* Most common type, involve the theme of being followed, harassed, cheated, poisoned or drugged, conspired against, attacked or harmed (by poisoning or plotting to murder) or spied on by extraordinary gadgets like radio-imaging or computer-assisted microwave monitoring or leaser photography, etc. or obstructed in the pursuit of goals by a person or group of persons.
  - *Querulous or litigious paranoia:* Manifested in querulant behavior. A querulant (meaning 'complaining') is a person who obsessively feels wronged, particularly about minor causes of action and they usually repeatedly petition authorities or pursue legal actions based on manifestly unfounded or too trivial grounds. Currently, this term is rarely used.
  - *Delusions of reference:* Casual events have a special, usually dangerous, significance in reference to him/her (other persons are talking about him/people on television or radio are talking about him, or headlines or stories in newspapers are written especially for them).
  - *Delusions of control or influence or passivity:* Some outside force or agency is controlling thoughts and feelings. Common symptoms are *thought broadcasting-* private thoughts are being transmitted to others; *thought insertion*—someone is planting thoughts into patient's head and *thought withdrawal*— Federal Bureau of Investigation (FBI) or police is robbing his/her own thoughts.
  - *Delusion of mind being read:* Other people can know one's thoughts. This is different from thought broadcasting in that the person does not believe that his or her thoughts are heard aloud.
  - *Delusions of jealousy or infidelity:* A belief that one's spouse is unfaithful, despite no supporting evidence. Commoner in men with alcohol problems and is associated with a risk of violence.

- **Somatic delusions**: Usually these are of three main types:
  1. *Delusion of infestation or delusional parasitosis (Ekbom's syndrome):* Patient believes that insects or worms or animals are infesting the skin or body. Usually, the imaginary parasites are reported as being "bugs" or insects crawling on or under the skin; the experience of this sensation is called formication. Karl Axel Ekbon (1907–1977) a Swedish neurologist published seminal account on this in 1937–38. The term "delusions of parasitosis" was introduced in 1946 by Wilson and Miller.
  2. *Delusions of dysmorphophobia:* Patient believes that he/she is having an ugly look or defective/abnormal size of body parts.
  3. *Delusion of foul body odors (Halitosis):* Patient believes he/she is having foul body odor, also known as olfactory reference syndrome.
- **Grandiose delusions:** Belief that one has special powers and is accomplishing or will accomplish extraordinary things for good of the community. Grandiose delusions are characterized by profound beliefs that one is famous, having special powers or ability (e.g. communicating with deceased relatives or extraterrestrial), omnipotent, often with a supernatural, science-fictional or religious bent. Usually, an elaborate loosely formed plan or program of activity is attached to this delusion.
- **Religious delusions:** Any delusion with a religious or spiritual content. A belief that one has a special power of God or God-like and has sacred duties towards mankind or chosen by God. Beliefs that would be considered normal for an individual's religious or cultural background are not delusions.
- **Technological delusions:** Patient believes that he/she is somehow connected to computers or other extraordinary (electrical or magnetic) gadgets, allowing him/her to exert immense power (one pt said by this power he may "create chaos in the cosmos").
- **Other delusions:**
  - *Erotic or amorous delusion (de Clerembault's syndrome):* Patient believes another person, usually of higher social status and standing, is secretly in love with the patient and communicates this in oblique ways. This was described by Gaëtan Gatian de Clérambault (2.7.1872–17.11.1934), a French psychiatrist, in his publication of *Les Psychoses Passionelles* in 1921.
  - *Nihilistic delusion (Cotard's syndrome):* Patient thinks that internal organs have disappeared or rotted away or the family, possessions or even the whole world has been destroyed or disappeared, or things (or everything, including the self) do not exist; a sense that everything is unreal. This syndrome was first described by Jules Cotard (1.6.1840-19.8.1889), a French neurologist.
  - *Delusion of guilt or sin (delusion of self-accusation):* Patient thinks they are guilty of any minor or imagined behavior or event that may be related or unrelated with him/her.
  - *Delusion of poverty*: A false belief that one is impoverished or will be deprived of material possessions. Depressed patients are prone to *delusions of poverty* and *delusions of nihilism*. The future is hopeless, the present desolate, the patient destitute

and abandoned to a bleak fate. Depressed patients may also suffer from inordinate *guilt*, the most extreme punishments being meted out to them for unremarkable, ancient transgressions.
- *Hypochondriacal delusion*: These are false beliefs about illness. Despite effective medical evidence to the contrary, the patient believes that he/she is suffering from serious diseases. Commonly seen in delusional disorder, depression and schizophrenia.

- **Delusional misidentification syndrome**: It is an umbrella term, introduced by Christodoulou (1986) for a group of delusional beliefs that occur in the context of psychiatric or neurological disorders. They core delusional belief is relating to the changed or altered identity of a person, object or place. As these delusions typically only concern one particular topic, they are also called monothematic delusions.
  - *Capgras delusion:* The belief that a close relative or spouse has been replaced by an identical-looking impostor. First reported in 1923 by Capgras and Reboul-Lachaux. Joseph Capgras (1873–1950) was a French psychiatrist, and J Reboul-Lachaux was his intern. They named it as "Illusions of double".
  - *Reverse Capgras*: The patient believes others think he is an imposter.
  - *Fregoli delusion*: The belief that different people are in fact a single person who changes appearance or is in disguise. This was named after the famous Italian stage actor Leopold Fregoli (2.7.1867-26.11.1936) who had extraordinary ability in impersonations and his quickness in exchanging roles. P Courbon and G Fail first reported the condition in 1927 (Ellis et al. 1994).
  - *Reverse Fregoli delusion*: The patient believes that he looks like a famous person.
  - *Intermetamorphosis:* The belief that people in one's environment swap identities with each other whilst maintaining the same appearance, so that A becomes B, B becomes C and so on. P Courbon and J Tusques reported this in 1932 (Ellis et al. 1994).
  - *Subjective doubles* (*Christodoulou, 1978*): The delusion belief that the person has a double or doppelganger with the same appearance, but usually with different character traits and leading a life of its own. Sometimes the patient has the idea that there is more than one double.
  - *Mirrored self-misidentification*: The belief that one's reflection is of another person. A related rare phenomenon is 'negative autoscopy', characterized by the failure to perceive one's mirror image while looking into a mirror, often found in dementia, traumatic brain injury or neurological illness (Dening and Berrios, 1994).
  - *Reduplicative paramnesia*: Characterized by the belief that a familiar person, place, object or body part is believed duplicated, existing in two or more places simultaneously, e.g. the patient thinks his real home has been moved and that he is living in an identical looking home (Taylor and Vaidya, 2009). This term was used first by Czech neurologist Arnold Pick in 1903.
  - *Delusional companions*: It is characterized by the belief that certain non-living objects (like toys) possess consciousness and can think independently and feel emotion. This belief is transient and normal in childhood but abnormal in an adult.

- *Clonal pluralization of self:* Characterized by the belief that he/she exists in plural numbers—there are many physically and psychologically identical copies of a given original (Voros et al. 2003).
- **Communicated delusions**: It is seen in couples (folie à deux) or in families (folie à famille)— usually, there is one dominant member who induced the delusion in the passive partner or other members.
    - *Folie à deux (madness for two) or Folie impose*: Also called induced psychosis, is a delusional disorder shared by two or more people (folie à plusieurs) who are closely related emotionally. One suffers from 'real' psychosis while the symptoms of psychosis are induced in the other or others, due to close attachment to the one with psychosis. Separation usually results in symptomatic improvement in the one who is not psychotic.
    - *Folie simultanée*: A delusional system emerges simultaneously and independently in two closely related persons, and the separation of the two would not be beneficial in the resolution of psychopathology.
    - *Folie communiqué*: Occurs when a normal person suffers a contagion of his ideas after resisting them for a long time. Once he acquires these beliefs, he maintains them despite the separation.
    - *Folie induite*: A person who is already psychotic, adds the delusions of a closely associated person to his own.

    Shared or mass delusion: Spontaneous, en masse development of an irrational belief leading to identical physical or emotional symptoms among a group of individuals (usually as a reaction to a recent event). Also known as collective hysteria, epidemic hysteria, mass psychogenic illness. It is the operative force in psychiatric epidemics Koro (Chowdhury, 2015), penis loss, fainting/dancing epidemics.

    DSM-5 removed the distinction between delusional disorder and shared delusional disorder, in which two or more individuals share a delusional belief, historically referred to as folie à deux.
- **Pseudocyesis or 'false pregnancy' or 'phantom pregnancy':** Is a state when a non-pregnant woman has a false belief that she is pregnant and presents marked bodily signs of pregnancy (i.e. amenorrhea, breast changes, nausea, abdominal enlargement, reported fetal movements, weight gain, etc.). It usually occurs in hysterical women with infantile personalities and abnormal sexual histories, also when a woman is either desperate for a child or is overwhelmed by fears that she may be pregnant or in relation to infertility in women with normal sexual behavior. Pseudocyesis can be delusional when the false belief of pregnancy is firm and unshakable. Pseudocyesis and delusional pregnancy can be differentiated by the absence or presence of somatic manifestations of the gravid state.
- **Delusion of pregnancy:** It is a special form of hypochondriacal/somatic delusion. It is nosologically nonspecific, occurring in schizophrenia and schizo-affective disorder, delusional disorders, affective disorders, epilepsy, dementia, and other organic brain syndromes, as well as in medical conditions like urinary tract infection, drug-induced lactation, and polydipsia and hyponatremia syndrome (Simon et al. 2009). Delusion of

pregnancy in male and animal pregnancy in male as a culture-bound syndrome has been reported (Chowdhury, 2003).

[*Couvade syndrome:* The father of the child to be born mimics the behavior of his pregnant wife in labor. Husband displays different somatic symptoms of pregnancy. It is a type of conversion symptom where husband's anxiety over his wife's gravid state manifests in somatic symptoms. It is not delusional as the husband does not believe himself to be pregnant. It has a strong cultural connection.]

- **Delusion of rape:** It represents a complex mixture of delusional belief and somatic delusion (of genital penetration), usually complained that occurred during sleep by schizophrenic female patients.
- **Delusion of sex change:** Delusions of sex change is not uncommon in body dysmorphic disorder and schizophrenia (especially paranoid type). Coexisting of transsexualism and schizophrenia sometimes cause a lot of clinical confusion in the differential diagnosis of gender identity disorder and psychosis (Urban and Rabe-Jablonska, 2010; Kowalczyk, 2015). Recently, a female case of delusion of sex change in the postictal phase of partial epilepsy with an amygdale tumor is reported and diagnosed as 'ictal delusional misidentification syndrome' (Kasper et al. 2009).
- **Bizarre and non-bizarre delusion:** Categorization of delusion on the basis of content as Bizarre and Non-bizarre is important from the diagnostic point of view. DSM IV considered the presence of bizarre delusion as one of the criteria in the diagnosis of schizophrenia so long as dysfunction/suffering and length-of-illness criteria are satisfied (Cermolacce et al. 2010). The concept of bizarreness is defined in DSMs through the following notions (Cermolacce et al. 2010) as (a.) physical (or perhaps logical) impossibility, (b.) generally not shared in cultural context, and (c.) overall implausibility or incomprehensibility with emphasis on grounding in ordinary experience, although some authors have raised the issue of reliability (Mojtabi and Nichilson, 1995) and validity (Nakaya et al. 2002) of bizarre delusion as diagnostic criteria (Flaum et al. 1991) for schizophrenia.

Non-bizarre delusion is considered as diagnostic for delusional disorder. Non-bizarre delusions, in contrast to bizarre delusions, are those delusions that reflect real-life situations (which, though false belief, is at least possible or could be true) and may include feelings of being followed, poisoned, infected, deceived or conspired against, or loved at a distance. The diagnostic criteria include the following: Non-bizarre delusion for at least one month, absence of odd or bizarre delusion, never meet the criteria Schizophrenia, schizoaffective or mood disorder, absence of any organic pathology and absence of auditory or visual hallucinations for at least one week. Delusional disorders are subtyped into the following categories: Erotomanic type (Predominately erotomanic delusions); grandiose type (predominately grandiose delusions), jealous type (predominately delusions of jealousy), persecutory type (predominately persecutory delusions), somatic type (predominately somatic delusions) and unspecified type (Does not fit any of the previous categories).

DSM-5 changes the diagnostic criteria for delusional disorder to reflect revision of the diagnostic criteria for schizophrenia. Mirroring the change in the schizophrenia diagnostic criteria, delusions in delusion disorder are no longer required to be of the "non-bizarre" type.

A person can now be diagnosed with delusional disorder with bizarre delusions, via a new specifier in the DSM-5.

- **Therianthropy:** Belief in a metamorphosis of humans into other animals. It is also known as 'Shapeshifting' that refers to an alteration of physical appearance, in this case, from human to animal. Lycanthropy (transformation into a wolf) is the most well-known form, followed by cynanthropy (transformation into a dog) and Ailuranthropy (transformation into a cat or feline). This has a strong relation with cultural folk myths and is now a rare psychiatric disorder (Chowdhury, 1992).

Culture and delusion: Our cultures provide the background material to understand the self and the environment, including the beliefs and the narrative for delusions. A good example is the extensive computer and internet use in recent decades—which is also incorporated in the delusional belief system (computer bug or cyber-spying). Cross-cultural studies suggest culture is intimately related to the delusional belief (Gaines, 1995). Studies also found that the general cultural beliefs, rather than the immediate environment, play a dominant role in determining the contents of delusion (Ahmed, 1978). A study among the psychotic patients showed that the delusion is a way of adaptation to stress specific to the culture, rather than as wish-fulfilling fantasies, denials, or projections derived from internal conflicts (Roy, 1962). Sharing of beliefs among society in mass delusion (in psychiatric epidemics) is a glaring example of the cultural root and its influence on the delusional content.

APPENDIX 17

Disorders of Perception

■ DISORDERS OF PERCEPTION

Perceptual Distortions

There is a *real* perceptual object but perceived in a distorted way. The common distortions are:
- *Changes in intensity*—perception may be altered; either heightened or diminished, e.g. Hyperacusis: Sounds of normal intensity are perceived as abnormally loud. Seen in migraine, hangover from alcohol excess, depressive disorders. Visual hyperesthesia: Colors look more intense or vivid. Seen in hypomania, epileptic aura, effect of lysergic acid diethylamide (LSD), and situations of intense emotion like religious fervor.
- *Changes in quality*—mainly visual perception are affected, brought about by toxic substances, e.g. coloring of yellow, green, or red, seen in mescaline or digitalis poisoning.
- *Changes in spatial form* (*Dysmegalopsia*)—an inability to judge the size or measure of an object accurately: Micropsia, macropsia, porropsia (visual distortion in which stationary objects appear to be moving away from the observer), metamorphosia. Seen in temporal and parietal lobe lesions, retinal disease, disorders of accommodation and convergence.
- *Distortion of experience of time*—There are two varieties of time: Physical and personal. It is the latter that is affected by psychiatric disorders, e.g. in severe depression patient may feel time passes slowly and even stands still. By contrast, the manic patient feels that time speeds by. However, the debate remains whether the perception of time is primarily a perceptual entity or has an added element of judgement.
- *Splitting of perception*—Changes in the emotional quality and associations of real percepts: Child during the early years splits his/her perception of mother as good or bad mother, and in time, that becomes the mental relationship that is reenacted in life relationships.

Perceptual Deceptions
- Illusions
- Hallucinations
- Distortions of body image (please see page 118)

Illusions

Illusions—misinterpretations of real sensory stimuli. An illusion may be:
- *Optical illusion*: It is characterized by visually perceived images that are deceptive or misleading
- *Auditory illusion*: It is an illusion of hearing. The listener hears either sounds which are not present in the stimulus, or "impossible" sounds
- *Tactile illusion* (e.g. phantom limb): It can occur with other senses including that of taste and smell
- *Completion illusion*: They depend on inattention for their occurrence, e.g. misreading words or missing misprints
- *Affect illusions*: They arise in the context of a particular mood state, e.g. a bereaved person may momentarily believe that they see the deceased person
- *Fantastic illusions* are perceived as extraordinary modifications of the environment. Frank Fish (2007) gave an example of one of his patients who, during an examination, saw Fish's head change into a rabbit's head
- *Muller–Lyer illusions* refer to perceptions that do not agree with the physical stimulus
- *Autokinetic illusion*: It is a visual perception in which there is an apparent movement of a stationary single point of light or small object at the background of a dark field when observed continuously. [A post-traumatic stress disorder (PTSD) patient after elephant attack perceived the change of head of the idol of Lord *Ganesh* during worship into a real moving elephant head, Chowdhury, 2014]
- *Eidetic image*: It is a vivid and detailed reproduction of a previous perception as in a "photographic memory"
- *Pareidolias*: It is playful, voluntary illusions from ambiguous or evanescent images, e.g. flames or clouds (without any conscious effort)
- *Trailing*: It is a visual illusion and it is the perception that an object moving steadily in space is followed by temporary, distinct after-images. Occur in fatigue, marijuana and mescaline intoxication.

Hallucination

A *hallucination* is a false perception that occurs in the waking state in the absence of a sensory stimulus. It is not merely a sensory distortion or misinterpretation but also carries a subjective sense of conviction. A true hallucination appears to the subject to be substantial and occurs in external objective space. In contrast, a mental imagery is insubstantial and experienced within an internal subjective space.

Hallucinatory experience may involve all the main sensory modalities, viz. olfactory, gustatory, visual, auditory and tactile. In addition, it may involve somatic (bodily) sensations, sexual sensations, vibrations, sensation of heat and cold, kinesthetic and proprioceptive sensations and the experience of time. The historical tripartite division of the hallucination states three groupings; dreams, delirium and hallucination proper (Berrios and Porter, 1999). Depending on the modalities involved, hallucinations can be grouped as:

Elementary hallucinations are simple phenomena that confine themselves to a single sensory modality.

Organized hallucinations are more complex in nature, ranging from simple geometrical patterns (or tunes, in the auditory modality) to full-color, three-dimensional images (or symphonies), within a single sensory modality.

Complex hallucination is used to denote hallucinated symphonies, three-dimensional images, occurring in more than one sensory modality. Often referred to as compound or multimodal hallucinations.

Hallucinosis: It is a pathologic mental state in which awareness consists primarily or exclusively of hallucinations, not associated with clouding of consciousness (e.g. alcoholic hallucinosis, organic hallucinosis in dementia). Sensory deprivation may produce visual and auditory hallucinosis in many subjects. Hallucinosis and delirium (for e.g. following cataract surgery) probably act by the same mechanism, especially in association with dementia. Diencephalic and cortical disease may be associated with hallucinations (usually visual). Tumors of the olfactory or basal temporal regions may cause olfactory hallucinosis, for example, like an aura.

Box 1: History.

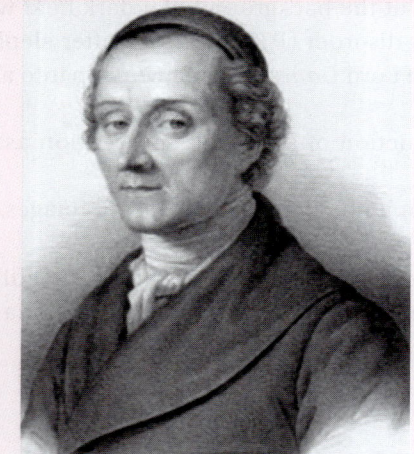
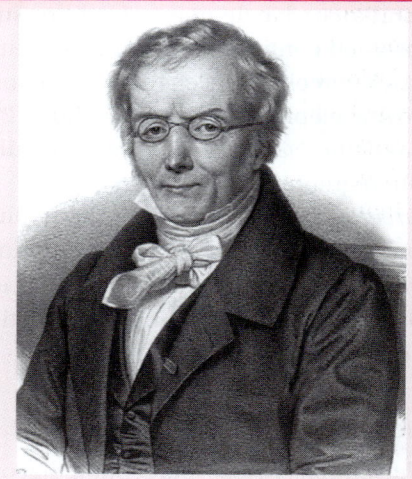

Johann Kaspar Lavater
(15.11.1741–02.01.1801)

Esquirol
(04.01.1772–12.12.1840)

The word "hallucinatory" has its roots in the Latin *hallucinari* or *allucinari*, which means to *wander in mind*. Lavater, a Swiss poet and physiognomist, introduced "hallucination" in the English language in 1572 to refer to "ghosts and spirits walking the night". The word was first used in its current sense in 1837 by Jean-Etienne Dominique Esquirol, a French psychiatrist.

In the middle ages, hallucinations were thought to be manifestations of demons or angels. A religious person who experienced such phenomena was seen as a saint, whereas a commoner was believed to be possessed by the devil. In certain cultures, hallucinations are still perceived as the work of Satan or as a result of magic (Wahass & Kent, 1997).

Types of Hallucinations
1. **Auditory hallucination**: It is false perception of sound, usually voices but also other noises such as music. Most common hallucination in psychiatric disorders. It is also known as *Paracusia*. The most common type of auditory hallucinations in psychiatric illness consists of voices; that is verbal hallucination. Voices may be male or female, usually hear more than one voice, and these are sometimes recognized as belonging to someone who is familiar (such as a neighbor, family member, or TV personality) or to an imaginary character (God, the devil, spirits, an angel). Verbal hallucinations may comprise full sentences but may be of single words. The lack of voluntary control over the experience is a key feature of auditory hallucinations.

Command hallucination: An auditory hallucination of a commanding voice, instructing or ordering the patient to perform a particular action. Also known as teleological hallucination.

Imperative hallucination: A type of command hallucination in which the hallucinatory instruction is experienced as irresistible, a combination of command hallucination and passivity action.

2. **Visual hallucination**: It is false perception involving sight consisting of both formed images (people, animal, insect) and unformed or elemental images (flashes of light or color). In general, visual hallucination suggests acute brain disorder and tends to occur in a setting of confusion or obtundation. In delirium, insects or other small objects may be seen moving on the bed. Lilliputian hallucinations, of little people on the bed, may occur in delirium and other organic brain syndromes.

Peduncular hallucinosis, first described by J Lhermitte in 1922, is a rare form of visual hallucinations most commonly caused by lesions to the midbrain and thalamus or by other neurological diseases like multiple sclerosis in which the person has vivid, colorful, or distorted images of animals and people. They are considered nonthreatening by the patient.

Anton's syndrome, a form of cortical blindness, in which patients deny their blindness despite objective evidence of visual loss, and moreover confabulate to support their stance. They may have other injury to the occipital cortex or other cortical centers, but the patients typically behave as if they were sighted.

Complex audiovisual hallucinations may occur in temporal lobe epilepsy. Sometimes, however, a schizophrenic patient may report visual hallucinations (e.g. trips in flying saucers) aligned with his/her prevailing delusions. The visual hallucinations of hysteria or dissociative disorder have a pseudohallucinatory quality and sometimes represent a past-traumatic event.

Features of visual hallucinations (adopted from Teeple et al. 2009)

Clinical picture of visual hallucination	Probable etiology
Simple pattern like spots, flashing shapes or lines, usually unilateral distribution, associated with headache	Migraine (aura of migraine), seizure, brain tumor (that lie along or compress the optic path)

Contd...

Contd...

Clinical picture of visual hallucination	Probable etiology
Macropsia, micropsia, metamorphopsia a distorted vision due to macular pathology, in which lines appear wavy, parts of the line appear blank and flat surface bend (a patient may see a tree bending despite the fact that it is straight)	Seizure, Creutzfeldt-Jacob disease
Related with onset to or waking from sleep	Hypnagogic or hypnopompic hallucination
Confabulation with anosognosia	Anton's syndrome
Frightening content	Psychotic disorder (schizophrenia, schizoaffective disorder, bipolar disorder, major depressive disorder), delirium, hallucinogenic drug
Good insight	Charles Bonnet syndrome, migraine, peduncular hallucinosis

3. ***Olfactory hallucination (Phantosmia)***—false perception of smell, most common in medical disorder (e.g. smell of burning rubber, steak and onions may occur in temporal lobe epilepsy. Schizophrenic patients may perceive the odor of gas being pumped into their bedrooms by persecutors). *Parosmia*, smell is actually present but perceived differently from its usual smell.

4. ***Gustatory hallucination***—false perception of taste such as unpleasant taste, caused by uncinate fits of complex partial seizure. A schizophrenic patient may think they taste poisonous substances in their food. *Phantageusia* is a sudden, vague taste without the presence of the substance normally causing the sensation. Olfactory and gustatory hallucinations most often associated with organic brain diseases, particularly with the uncinate fits of complex partial seizures.

5. ***Somatic (Hallucination of bodily sensation)***—a hallucination involving the perception of a physical experience occurring within the body, i.e. perception of things occurring in or to the body, most often of visceral origin (also called Cenesthetic hallucination). Somatic hallucinations occur in schizophrenia, where genital, visceral, intracerebral or kinesthetic sensations are often referred to being the influence of persecutors or machines. A depressed patient may have the sense of having no stomach, with food dropping from the throat into a void.

Kinesthetic or proprioceptive hallucination—a hallucination involving the sense of bodily movement like feeling that limbs are twisted or sense of altered posture (sensations as floating, flying or having out-of-body experience). German psychiatrist August Cramer (1860–1912) published the first clinical study on kinesthetic hallucination in 1889.

Haptic or tactile hallucination—false perception of touch or surface sensation as from an amputated limb (phantom limb) or crawling sensation over or under the skin (**formication** in alcohol withdrawal syndrome, cocaine intoxication). May be associated with delusion of **parasitosis**. Some tactile hallucinations like having intercourse with a deity or some other particular alleged person (**sexual hallucinations**—erection, orgasm, and penetration) are highly suggestive of schizophrenia. Thermic (abnormal perception of heat and cold 'feet are on fire') and hygric (a perception of fluid feeling of 'water running on the chest') hallucinations are seen in psychosis.

Proprioceptive hallucinations—it is the hallucination of body posture; where the individual experiences sensations such as floating, flying or having an out-of-body experience. The person may describe the sensation that a part of his/her body part is at a different location (e.g. phantom limbs). The term 'proprioception' (perceiving one's own position) was coined by British neurophysiologist Charles Scott Sherrington (1857–1952).

6. ***Autoscopic hallucination (phantom mirror image)***—hallucinations of one's own physical self; experience of seeing one's own body projected into external space, usually in front of oneself for short periods. This term was first used by C Fere in 1891. This may stimulate the delusion that one has a double. In **internal autoscopy,** the subject sees his or her own internal organs. In **negative autoscopy,** the patient looks at the mirror and sees no image at all. Seen in acute and subacute delirious state, epilepsy, focal lesions affecting parietal-occipital regions. Reported in near-death and out-of-body experiences of hospitalized subjects.

7. ***Functional hallucinations***—hallucinations in which the person experiences auditory hallucinations simultaneously through another real noise (i.e. in the same sensory modality), e.g. a sound of running water triggers a hallucinatory voice or a person perceive auditory hallucination only when he hears a car engine or pattering raindrops. Very often found in delirium and toxic states, seizure disorder and focal brain vascular disease.

8. ***Reflex hallucinations***—a stimulus in one sensory field leads to a hallucination in another, e.g. a schizophrenic patient would feel a sharp chest pain every time a certain family member called his name. It is a form of synesthesia.

9. ***Extracampine hallucinations***—hallucination that occurs outside the patient's sensory field, e.g. a young schizophrenic patient hearing verbal command of Bill Clinton in USA from India.

10 ***Musical hallucination***—a form of auditory hallucination in which music is heard, often the same piece of music. In most cases, the music is familiar to the person. It is most common in older people, especially women, with hearing loss. It is suggested that sensory deprivation from the deafness is the cause. It may also result from specific lesions in the dorsal pons, brain tumor or abscess and epileptic activity. It is also reported from patients with depression, obsessive-compulsive disorder (OCD), schizophrenia and alcoholism.

11 ***Synesthesia***—stimulation of one sensory modality evokes perceptual distortions in another as if sensory modalities seem fused, e.g. sound seen or colors felt. Found in marijuana and mescaline intoxication, also a normal experience in many people.

12 ***Migrainous hallucinations***—reported by 50% of patients with migraine; visual hallucinations of geometric patterns, sometimes with micropsia and macropsia. Also known as the Alice in Wonderland syndrome.

13 ***Ictal hallucinations***—occurring as a part of seizure activity, typically brief and stereotyped, in a state of altered consciousness or a twilight sleep.

14 ***Hypnagogic***—false sensory perception occurring while falling asleep, generally considered nonpathological. Severe sleep deprivation can cause hypnagogic hallucination.

15 ***Hypnopompic***—false sensory perception occurring while awakening from sleep, generally considered nonpathological. Both occur in healthy people and are characteristic symptoms of narcolepsy.

16 ***Mood congruent***—hallucinatory content is consistent with either a depressed or manic mood.

17 ***Mood incongruent***—hallucinatory content is not consistent with either a depressed or manic mood.

18 ***Pseudohallucinations***—perceptions experienced as coming from within the mind (vivid images that are heard or seen from within; Jasper, 1911). Obsessional ruminations or intrapsychic self-reproach in severe depressive guilt are sometimes expressed as "voices". Frequently found in borderline personality disorder cases.

19 ***Experiential hallucinations***—the term coined by Canadian neurosurgeon Wilder Graves Penfield (1891–1976) and defined as "hallucinations made up of elements from the individual's past experiences. They may seem to him so strange that he calls them dreams, but when they are carefully analyzed, it is evident that the hallucination is a shorter or longer sequence of past experience. *The subject relives a period of the past although he is still aware of the present."*

20 ***Panoramic hallucination***—it is also known as scenic or holocampine hallucination which denotes a compound hallucination in which the entire sensory input is replaced by hallucinatory percepts, thus giving rise to a totally different perceptual reality. It is similar to experiential hallucination and is usually found in temporal lobe psychosensory epilepsy, delirium and PTSD flashbacks.

21 ***Flashback***—an intense visual reexperience of highly charged past events, which are often replays of hallucinations. These images are usually triggered by a trivial reminder of the past experiences (e.g. a smell or sound) and usually brief and intensely upsetting. Typically seen in LSD and mescaline use, in PTSD.

22 **Delusional perception**—a true perception, to which a patient attributes a false meaning. For example, a perfectly normal event such as the traffic lights turning red may be interpreted by the patient as meaning that the aliens are about to land. It is one of Schneider's first rank symptoms. Though it is highly indicative of schizophrenia, it can also occur in other psychoses, including mania with grandiose color.

23. **Charles Bonnet syndrome**—patients who are visually impaired often develop pseudohallucinations (visual hallucinations) with preserved cognitive status. A similar phenomenon is the musical hallucination in individuals with acquired deafness.

> **Box 2:** Charles Bonnet (13.03.1720–20.05.1793).
>
>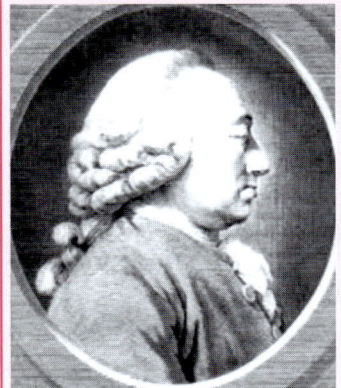
>
> A Swiss naturalist and philosophical writer. In 1760, he described a condition now called **Charles Bonnet Syndrome** in which vivid, complex visual hallucinations (fictive visual percepts) occur in psychologically normal people. He documented it in his 87-year-old grandfather, who was nearly blind from cataracts in both eyes but perceived men, women, birds, carriages, buildings, tapestries and scaffolding patterns. Most people affected are elderly with visual impairments. However, the phenomenon does not occur only in the elderly or in those with visual impairments; it can also be caused by damage elsewhere in their optic pathway or brain.

Some Clinical Features of Auditory Hallucination

Auditory Hallucinations in Schizophrenia

These are usually of five types:
1. Audible thoughts described as hallucinated voices that speak aloud what the patient is thinking (*echo de la pensee*)
2. Voices that give a running commentary on the patient's actions
3. Hearing two or more voices arguing with each other, often about the patient who is referred to in the third person
4. Command hallucination—order patients to do things
5. Various meaningless sounds, e.g. buzzes, hums or rumbles.

Second person hallucinations—a voice appears to address the patient in the second person e.g. the voice may be talking directly to the patient; "You are going to die"; or the voice may direct the patient to do some action; "kill him". These types of auditory hallucinations are not diagnostic in the same way as third person auditory hallucinations, but the content of the hallucination and the patient's reaction to it may help the diagnosis.

Third person hallucinations—patients hear voices talking about themselves, referring to them in the third person, for example, "he is a bad person". This type of auditory hallucination is particularly associated with schizophrenia but can occur in affective disorders. Such voices may be experienced as commenting on the patient's intended actions like; "he wants to kill her", or describing his current actions; "he is trying to sleep now". A running commentary by voices is most suggestive of schizophrenia.

Voices or Phoneme—phoneme is a term from linguistics, which denotes the set of speech sounds in any given language. German neuropathologist Carl Wernicke (15.05.1848–15.06.1905) used this term to designate hallucinated voices in 1900. It is also known as verbal auditory hallucination (VAH) that is primarily verbal in nature and different from other auditory hallucinations (e.g. musical hallucination or nonverbal auditory hallucinations (Sommer et al. 2003). Phonemes are the most common form of hallucinations in patients with manic-depressive illness and schizophrenia. Voices may have the following character:

- May consist of one or more voices
- Frequency—intermittent or constant, whether related to any specific situation, location or activity
- *Type of Voice*—may be heard in a regular tone of voice, whisper or a shout, may be intelligible or unintelligible, may be clear or vague and may speak in a foreign language. It may be **Inchoate** (e.g. humming, rushing water, inaudible murmurs) or **Fragmentary** (e.g. words or phrases such as "fag", "get him," or "beastly") or **Complex,** typically, a schizophrenic patient identifies complex hallucinations in inner or outer space, as a voice or voices speaking to or about him/her
- *Source*—may be perceived as coming from within the head or other body parts like the abdomen (internal auditory hallucination) or from outside the head (external auditory hallucination) or may be swapping the location. They may be perceived as originating from alleged implants (e.g. transmitter or camera in the brain) or electronic devices like television or radio or from nearby locations (from outside the window), or even from a distant place or from space
- *Nature*—voices may be benign (they may give valuable advice or make pleasant comments) or malignant (insulting and threatening). When they consist of spoken orders or incentives, they are referred to as **command hallucinations**. They may also give **a running commentary** on the individual's thoughts or behavior
- *Content of voices*—varies between individuals. Often the voices have a negative and malicious content. They might speak in a derogatory or insulting manner or give commands to perform an unacceptable behavior. The experience of negative voices causes considerable distress. They may be positive or neutral.

Descriptive Features of Auditory Verbal Hallucination

Laroi et al. 2012 provided an excellent clinical analysis of Auditory-Verbal hallucinations (AVH) in schizophrenia and stressed the following descriptive features as a part of clinical examination in schizophrenia:

- Acoustic properties (verbal, nonverbal, loudness, clarity)
- Linguistic properties varies as low linguistic complexity (hearing words), medium (hearing sentences), high complexity (hearing conversations)
- Frequency (ranging from once or twice weekly to almost continuous)
- Control (lack of perceived control)
- Inner-outer localization (experienced as coming from inside the head or outside the head)

- Content (often comprised of commands, personal insults, and abuse, although they may also be positive or neutral)
- Personification (male or female; young or old)
- Appraisals (different explanations and attributions, e.g. forces of Good or Evil; conspiracy or plot; ghosts, spirits, or aliens).

Schneider's First Rank Symptoms in Schizophrenia

The first-rank symptoms (FRS) are a group of 11 symptoms which are important in the diagnosis of schizophrenia. Studies (Thorup et al. 2007) showed that approximately half of the patients with schizophrenia experience these symptoms. These are as follows:
- *Auditory hallucinations:*
  - Third-person auditory hallucinations discussing or arguing about the patient
  - Thought echo (audible thoughts)
  - Running commentary of patient's actions.
- *Delusions of thought interference:*
  - Thought insertion, withdrawal or broadcast.
- *Delusion of control:*
  - Somatic passivity (delusional belief that one is a passive recipient of bodily sensations from an external agency)
  - Passivity of impulse, affect and volition (made impulse, affect and volition).
- *Delusional perception:*
  - Delusional perception (a normal perception is suddenly interpreted in a delusional manner).

Auditory Hallucinations, Broadcasting of Thought, Controlled Thought (Delusions of Control), Delusional Perception (ABCD)

The reliability of using FRS for the diagnosis of schizophrenia has since been questioned, although the terms might still be used descriptively by mental health professionals who do not use them as diagnostic aids. FRS is not exclusive to schizophrenia; it also occurs in patients with manic-depressive illness, delirium or intoxication, dementia, seizure disorder, and stroke. Individuals with dissociative identity disorder (DID) may experience FRS more commonly than even patients with schizophrenia though patients with DID lack negative symptoms of schizophrenia and normally do not mistake hallucinations for reality.

> **Box 3:** Kurt Schneider (07.01.1887–27.10.1967).
>
> A German psychiatrist known largely for his writing on the diagnosis and understanding of Schizophrenia, as well as personality disorder, then known as psychopathic personalities. Schneider coined the terms **endogenous depression**, derived from Emil Kraepelin's use of the adjective to mean biological in origin, and **reactive depression**, usually often seen in outpatients, in the 1920s. Schneider also played a key role in developing concepts of psychopathy, used in a broad sense to mean personality disorder or particularly antisocial personality disorder. He published the influential **"The Psychopathic Personalities"** in 1923. This was based in part on his earlier 1921 work "The Personality and Fate of Registered Prostitutes" where he outlined 12 character types.

Frequency of Hallucinations (Yager and Gitlin, 2004)
- 10–27% of the general population have visual hallucination
- 50% grieving spouses have auditory or visual hallucinations
- 90% of patients with hallucinations also have delusions
- 35% of patients with delusions also have hallucinations
- 60–90% patients of schizophrenia have auditory hallucinations
- 20% manic patients have auditory hallucinations
- 10% of depressed patients experience auditory hallucination.

Cross-cultural explanation: Research (Al-Issa, 1995) shows that there are some cultural differences in the content and interpretation of voices. Auditory hallucinations occur in similar forms in all societies, but in cultures where they are understood in the context of local beliefs and practices, auditory hallucinations have a positive value.

Laroi et al. 2014 stated that hallucination has different patterns among clinical and nonclinical population. Culture influence the meaning and characteristics of hallucination associated with psychosis. Cultural variations have implication for the clinical outcome in psychosis. They concluded that "a clinician should never assume that the mere report of what seems to be hallucination is necessarily a symptom of pathology and that the patient's cultural background needs to be taken into account when assessing and treating hallucinations".

Causes of Hallucinations
- **Psychotomimetic drugs**—also called hallucinogenic, causing alteration of consciousness, e.g. Ecstasy (3,4-methylenedioxymethamphetamine, or MDMA), LSD, mescaline (3,4,5-trimethoxyphenethylamine, or peyote), and psilocybin (4-phosphoryloxy-N, N-dimethyltryptamine, or mushrooms), amphetamine, cannabis. Alcohol withdrawal may induce tactile and visual hallucinations (delirium tremens); haptic (tactile) hallucinations and formication (ants crawling) caused by cocaine, and hygric (feeling of water) hallucination occur with LSD.
- **Disorders of central negative system**—lesions of the cortex produce hallucinations, depending on the site of lesion (visual cortex → visual hallucination). In epilepsy, hallucinations of all sensory modalities are seen. A hallucinatory sensation, usually involving touch (an aura), often appears before a migraine attack.
- **Sensory deprivation/sleep deprivation or exhaustion**—physical and emotional exhaustion can induce hallucinations by blurring the line between sleep and wakefulness.
- **Hypnosis and trance state**—hallucinations are induced by strong suggestion.
- **Emotions**—in depression with guilt and self-reproach. Up to 75% of schizophrenic patients admitted for treatment report hallucinations.
- **Organic brain conditions** such as delirium, toxic and metabolic encephalopathies. Brain damage or injuries may produce hallucinations.
- **Stress**—prolonged and extreme stress/physical exhaustion can impede thought processes and trigger hallucinations.

- **Electrical or neurochemical activity in the brain**—a hallucinatory sensation, usually involving touch (an aura), often appears before a migraine attack. Auras involving smell and touch (tactile) are known to precede the onset of an epileptic attack.

Conditions Simulating Hallucinations
- After images (positive or negative)
- Eidetic images (photographic image)—ability to retain the image of an original stimulus in all clarity, detailed and vividness even after the stimulus is removed, can be recalled after a long time.
- Memory images (Imagery)—vivid visual experiences that can be produced and manipulated voluntarily (in trance state), product of own imagination, occur in the internal objective space, under the control of will.

Fake Hallucinations (Resnick and Knoll, 2005)
Malingered psychotic symptoms—detecting malingered mental illness is considered an advanced psychiatric skill. Malingerers may have inadequate or incomplete knowledge of the mental illness they are faking. Indeed, malingerers are like actors who can portray a role only as well as they understand it. They often overact their part or mistakenly believe the more bizarre their behavior, the more convincing they will be. Conversely, "successful" malingerers are more likely to endorse fewer symptoms and avoid endorsing overly bizarre or unusual symptoms. Numerous clinical factors suggest malingering. Malingerers are more likely to eagerly "thrust forward" their illness, whereas patients with genuine schizophrenia are often reluctant to discuss their symptoms. There must be a hidden agenda or goal behind the symptom presentation. Either to avoid some stressful situation like arrest, criminal prosecution or imminent joining a job or military or to seek controlled substances, compensation or disability benefits.

Some important points in the clinical examination are:
- **Hallucinations**—if a patient alleges atypical hallucinations, ask about them in detail. Hallucinations are usually (88%) associated with delusions (Lewinsohn, 1970). Genuine hallucinations are typically intermittent rather than continuous.
- **Auditory hallucinations**—are usually clear, not vague (7%) or inaudible. Both male and female voices are commonly heard (75%), and voices are usually perceived as originating outside the head (88%) (Goodwin et al. 1971). In Schizophrenia, the major themes are persecutory or instructive (Small et al. 1966). Comparing with the norm is another clinical way to identify fake hallucination (Rogers et al. 1984); 88% of real auditory hallucinations are from outside the head (usually outside the body or sometimes from a body part); 75% of real psychotics hear both male and female voices; 76% hear the hallucination in both ears, and 98% of hallucinations are spoken in the person's native language. Most auditory hallucinations are brief (<20 sec) and real psychotics can identify sex, race, age, and emotional state of the voice; the tone, volume, and rate of the voice and most auditory hallucinations ask for an interaction or a response from the person.

- ***Command auditory hallucinations***—are easy to fabricate. Persons experiencing genuine command hallucinations do not always obey the voices, especially if doing so would be dangerous and usually present with non-command hallucinations (85%) and delusions (75%) as well (Thompson et al. 1992). Solitary command hallucination without other psychotic symptoms raises the index of suspicion of malingering.
- ***Visual hallucinations*** are experienced by an estimated 24% to 30% of psychotic individuals but are reported much more often by malingerers (46%) than by persons with genuine psychosis (4%) (Cornell and Hawk, 1989). Genuine visual hallucinations are usually of normal sized people and are seen in color. On rare occasions, genuine visual hallucinations of small people (Lilliputian hallucinations) may be associated with alcohol use, organic disease, or toxic psychosis (such as anticholinergic toxicity) but are rarely seen by persons with schizophrenia. Psychotic visual hallucinations do not typically change if the eyes are closed or open, whereas drug-induced hallucinations are more readily seen with eyes closed or in the dark. Unformed hallucinations, such as flashes of light, shadows, or moving objects, are typically associated with neurologic disease and substance use. Suspect malingering if the patient reports dramatic or atypical visual hallucinations.

Appendix 18

Disorder of Identity and Will

Will—a goal-directed intention based on cognitively planned motivation.

Catatonic waxy flexibility—feeling of plastic resistance as the examiner moves the body and when the passive movement stops, the final posture is preserved.

Echolalia—psychopathological repetition of words or phrases of one person by another.

Echopraxia—pathological imitation of movements of one person by another.

Delusion of passivity—belief that own actions are controlled by some other being or agency.

Distortion of body image—misinterpretation of body sensation, anatomy or function. The term body image refers to the view that a person has of his or her own body size and proportion. Body-image distortion occurs when a person's view of their body is significantly different from reality as occurs in Anorexia nervosa or bulimia nervosa. *Dysmorphophobia* is the term used when there is an excessive dislike of a part of one's body. *Body dysmorphic disorder (BDD) is* characterized by excessive preoccupation with imagined defects in physical appearance. People with BDD are obsessed by the idea that some part of their body, their hair, nose, skin, hips, whatever, is ugly or deformed, when in truth it looks normal. They demand hormonal treatment or cosmetic or other surgery.

Dissociation—splitting of thoughts, feelings or behavior from everyday integrated conscious awareness.

Depersonalization—estrangement or detachment from a sense of personal existential presence.

Derealization—perception of the environment without a simultaneous feeling of conviction of its reality.

Dissociative amnesia—complete loss of memory and identity, but the subject can carry out complex patterns of behavior and is able to look after him so that there is a gross discrepancy between the marked memory loss and the intact personality.

Dissociative fugue—individual suddenly travels away from home, assumes a new identity and cannot recall important elements of his or her past life.

Unawareness of illness—truncated insight into psychiatrically determined disability ranging from inattention to complete denial.

Dissociative identity disorder (DID)—previously called multiple personality disorder; the diagnostic points are:
- The presence of two or more distinct identities, each with its own unique, and enduring, way of relating to the world and self
- At least two of these identities recurrently take control of the person's behavior
- An inability to recall important personal information to the extent that is more than ordinary forgetfulness, having a complete loss of memory for what happened in the previous few days.

Dissociative identity disorder (DID) would not be diagnosed if the symptoms did not cause a major disturbance to the person's life *or* if they were due to the physiological effects of a substance (e.g. drugs or alcohol) or a general medical condition.

Gender identity disorder—is characterized by strong, persistent cross-gender identification; with a strong belief that he/she is the victim of a biologic accident and are with a body incompatible with their subjective gender identity. Those with the most extreme form of the gender identity disorder are called transsexuals (Male-to-female transsexualism and Female-to-male transsexualism). These disorders are considered mental disorders because the body does not match the person's psychologic (felt) gender. Diagnosis rests on:
- Cross-gender identification (the desire to be or insistence that they are the other sex)
- A sense of discomfort about their sex or sense of substantial inappropriateness in their gender role
- Cross-gender identification must not be merely a desire for perceived cultural advantages of being the other sex
- There is significant distress or obvious impairment in social, occupational, or other important areas of functioning.

Cross-gender behavior, such as cross-dressing, may not require treatment if it occurs without concurrent psychologic distress or functional impairment or if a person has a physical intersex condition (e.g. congenital adrenal hyperplasia, ambiguous genitals, androgen insensitivity syndrome).

Distortions of body image—body image is a multifaceted cognitive construct involving perceptions, thoughts and feelings about one's physical being. It is the self-perception of appearance reflecting perceptual experience and subjective evaluation. The phrase "*body image*" was first coined by the Austrian psychiatrist and psychoanalyst Paul Ferdinand Schilder (15.02.1886–07.12.1940) in his book "*The Image and Appearance of the Human Body*" (1935). Body image distortions are an inaccurate perception of one's body shape, size or weight. Body dysmorphic disorder (BDD) is the extreme preoccupation and concern with body image, viz. a perceived defect in the physical appearance. In International Classification of Disease (ICD) 10, it bears the code F45.2 and placed under Somatoform disorder (F 45).

Several studies found abnormalities in different dimensions of body image in schizophrenia, viz. cognitive (thoughts, beliefs; body concept); affective (body satisfaction; body cathexis) and perceptual (body size estimation; body schema) (Chapman et al. 1978; Priebe and Rohricht, 2001).

Cenesthesias are abnormal body sensations and are not uncommon in schizophrenia. This term was coined by Johann Christain Reil (20.02.1759–22.11.1813), a German physician and psychiatrist who also coined the term "Psychiatry" 108 years ago. Patients with schizophrenia frequently report abnormal body sensations like sensations of pain, numbness, stiffness and feeling strange, abnormal heaviness, lightness, extension, diminution, shrinking, and enlargement of limbs, etc. (Rajender et al. 2009) and body experience like underestimation of lower extremities, desomatization, boundary loss and diminution (Rohricht and Priebe, 2002) and underestimation of body size (Kim et al. 2012). Varieties of disorders of body awareness-body schema disorder has been reported in the literature, mainly in the context organic brain pathology but some may be found in schizophrenic disorder (Barr, 1998) like phantom limb (perception of presence of amputated limb); macrosomatognosia (where either a part of the body, or the body as a whole, is experienced as disproportionally large-pathological accentuation of body image (may occur in hypochondriasis, depersonalization state, dissociative state, pseudocyesis, in dreams) and microsomatognosia (where the body, in part or in whole, is experienced as disproportionally small-diminished or absent body image). Usually, the last two types are associated with epileptic seizures, peripheral vascular disease, migraine, delirium, delirium tremens, alcohol withdrawal, mesencephalic lesions, and intoxication with hallucinogens such as LSD and mescaline.

Appendix 19

Attention and Concentration

Attention span—the amount of time that a person can concentrate on a task without becoming distracted.

Focused attention—the ability to respond discretely to specific visual, auditory or tactile stimuli.

Sustained attention (or vigilance)—the ability to maintain a consistent behavioral response during continuous and repetitive activity.

Selective attention—the ability to maintain a behavioral or cognitive set in the face of distracting or competing stimuli (freedom from distractibility).

Alternating attention—the ability of mental flexibility that allows individuals to shift their focus of attention and move between tasks having different cognitive requirements.

Divided attention—this is the highest level of attention, and it refers to the ability to respond simultaneously to multiple tasks or multiple task demands.

Distractibility—inability to concentrate attention; a state in which attention is drawn to unimportant or irrelevant external stimuli.

Hypervigilance—excessive attention and focus on all internal and external stimuli; usually secondary to delusional or paranoid states.

Trance—focused attention and altered consciousness, usually seen in hypnosis, dissociative disorders and ecstatic religious experiences.

Appendix 20

Memory

■ FUNCTIONS OF MEMORY

Registration—capacity to hold new information.

Retention—the ability to store information which can be returned to consciousness.

Retrieval—capacity to return stored material from memory.

Recall—the return of stored material to consciousness at a chosen moment.

Recognition—feeling familiarity when the stored material is returned to consciousness.

Forgetting (retention loss)—refers to apparent loss of information already encoded and stored in an individual's long-term memory. It is a spontaneous or gradual process in which old memories are unable to be recalled from memory storage.

■ TYPES OF MEMORY

Long-term memory or autobiographical memory—represent long-standing knowledge of our personal worlds; knowledge about self-development, family and childhood memories. Hyperthymestic syndrome—a rare condition where an individual has an extremely detailed autobiographical memory to recall specific events from his or her personal past.

Procedural memory or implicit memory—is not based on the conscious recall of information, but on implicit learning. It is primarily employed in learning motor skills.

Short-term memory or declarative or explicit memory—represents the new learning that goes on in our day-to-day lives. It has three components; episodic memory (memory of personally experienced events), semantic memory (memory of facts, principles and rules that make up general knowledge of the world) and emotional memory (contributes autonomic and emotional tone).

Topographic memory—is the ability to orient oneself in space, to recognize and follow an itinerary, or to recognize familiar places. Getting lost when traveling alone is an example of the failure of topographic memory, often reported among elderly dementia patients.

■ DISORDERS OF MEMORY

Amnesia—partial or total inability to recall past experiences. It may be psychological (dissociative amnesia) or organic (amnestic disorders).

Amnestic disorders are characterized by problems with memory function; either with difficulty in recalling events that happened or facts that were learnt before, called *retrograde amnesia* or with an inability to learn new facts or retain new memories, called *anterograde amnesia*. Amnestic disorders are caused by general medical conditions (e.g. head trauma, hypoxia, herpes simplex encephalitis, and posterior cerebral artery infarction) or substance use or accidental exposure to toxins. Alcohol abuse is a leading cause of substance-related amnestic disorder that leads to thiamine deficiency and induce Wernicke-Korsakoff's syndrome.

Wernicke's encephalopathy—a triad of symptoms; confusion, ataxia and eye signs (nystagmus or ophthalmoplegia) with profound inattentiveness, apathy and memory disorder.

Korsakoff's syndrome—dissociation between immediate recall and short-term memory with significant problems registering new information (anterograde amnesia) and also memory problems that predate the onset of the syndrome (retrograde amnesia).

Transient global amnesia—sudden onset of apparent confusion with loss of ability to learn new information; attacks last hours, rarely days and patients are concerned about their difficulties. Seen in complex partial seizures, migraine, and transient ischemia of the medial temporal lobes, sedative intoxication and cerebral neoplasm. Precipitating factors may include sudden alteration of body temperature or orgasm.

Traumatic amnesia—refers to a loss of memory both for a period of time preceding the head injury (retrograde amnesia) and for events following the injury (anterograde amnesia). It also prevents the registering of new information. Patients with bifrontal lesions may show *reduplicative paramnesia;* a delusion of being convinced that one is in a specific geographic location despite all evidence to the contrary.

Hypermnesia—exaggerated degree of retention and recall.

Paramnesia—disturbances of memory in which reality and fantasy are confused. Observed in dreams and in certain types of schizophrenia and organic mental disorders.
- Déjà vu—illusion of visual recognition in which a new situation is incorrectly regarded as a repetition of a previous experience
- Déjà entendu—illusion that what one is hearing, he has heard previously
- Déjà pense—condition in which a thought never entertained before is incorrectly regarded as a repetition of a previous experience
- Déjà eprouve—(already experienced, tested, tried out); deja fait (already done); deja raconte (already told, recounted) deja voulu (already desired)
- Jamais vu—a false feeling of unfamiliarity with a real situation that one has previously experienced.

Confabulation—unconscious filling of gaps in memory by imagining experiences or events that have no basis in reality, commonly seen in amnestic syndromes. Reflects frontal lobe dysfunction. Found in alcohol amnestic syndromes (Wernicke's-Korsakoff syndrome); disorders of mammillary bodies, thalamus or frontal lobe.

Perseveration—here the first response to a question is appropriate but inappropriate to the second stimulus, e.g. *First question*: Where you stay? The answer is Kolkata. *Second question*: How long you are here? The answer is Kolkata. It is a sign of organic brain disease.

Retrospective falsification—memory becomes unintentionally (unconsciously) distorted by being filtered through a person's present emotional, cognitive and experiential state.

Pseudologia fantastica—fluent untruthful statements, seen with hysterical behavior, malingering, and Munchausen syndrome (who feign disease or psychological trauma in order to draw attention or sympathy). Munchausen syndrome by proxy refers to the abuse of another being, typically a child, in order to seek attention or sympathy for the abuser).

Dementia is a syndrome, characterized by a decline in mental ability which affects memory, thinking, problem-solving, concentration and perception. Some forms of dementia, such as Alzheimer's disease, are degenerative while other like in vascular dementia, may be nondegenerative.

Psychogenic Memory Disturbances (Leung and Passmore, 2002)

- *Cryptamnesia*—failure to remember that one is remembering, e.g. believing that an argument is original when one has heard it from others before
- *Dissociative amnesia*—caused by trauma or stress, resulting in an inability to recall important personal information, not to be explained by normal forgetfulness.
- *Dissociative fugue*—sudden, unexpected travel away from home or one's customary place of work, with an inability to recall one's past with confusion about personal identity, or the assumption of a new identity
- *Approximate answers*—answering '7' when asked 'how much is 5 + 4'. Found in hysterical pseudodementia, some organic conditions and Ganser syndrome (a dissociative disorder)
- *Multiple personality disorder*—the apparent existence of two or more distinct personalities (with different memories, behaviors and preferences) within an individual, with only one being evident at any one time
- *Repressed memory or motivated forgetting*—used to describe a significant memory, usually of a traumatic nature, that has become unavailable for recall because the subject blocks out painful or traumatic times in one's life. Here both the process may be involved: Memories are dissociated from awareness as well as repressed without dissociation.

Clinical Significance and Test for Memory Disorders (Snyderman and Rovner, 2009)

Memory type	Clinical test	Deficit
Episodic: Ability to recall personal experiences	Knowing the breakfast menu/ how celebrated last birthday?	Transient in nature in seizure, concussion, amnesia, hypoglycemia, degenerative disorders, Alzheimer, dementia
Semantic: Ability to learn and store conceptual and factual information	Last Prime Minister of the country	Advanced Alzheimer disease
Procedural: Ability to learn behavioral/cognitive skills	Learning to ride a bike, swim	Parkinson disease, Huntington disease, cerebrovascular accidents (CVA), tumors
Working: Ability to maintain temporary information (combination of attention, concentration and short-term memory)	Remembering a phone number	Delirium

Appendix 21

Information and Intelligence

Learning disability: The World Health Organization (WHO) defines learning disabilities (LD) as "a state of arrested or incomplete development of mind" (Northfield, 2004). People with LD have significant impairment of intellectual functioning' and adaptive/social functioning. So, the person will have difficulties in understanding, learning and remembering new things. Difficulties with learning may lead to difficulties with a number of social tasks, for example, communication, self-care, awareness of health and safety. These impairments are present from childhood, not acquired as a result of an accident or following the onset of adult illness. There is still a debate about the best way to measure "significant" impairment and the impact of impairments of social functioning. Psychometric tests are usually used to measure intellectual functioning by measuring Intelligence Quotient (IQ). A common tool used to measure general intellectual functioning for the adult population is the Wechsler Adult Intelligence Scale (Wechsler, 1955). The mean of the scale is 100, and the standard deviation is 15. More than two standard deviations below the mean would suggest the presence of learning disability (hence IQ of 70 or less). IQ is used to classify the level of learning disability: Mild learning disability—IQ 50–70, Moderate—IQ 35–49, Severe—IQ 20–34 and Profound—IQ less than 20.

    Learning disability is a descriptive diagnosis or concept, not a disease or illness. It does not infer a particular etiology. Social functioning is an integral part of the diagnosis. It is important to understand that it is different from mental illness; a person with a learning disability can also develop mental illness. Learning disability as a concept is also different from "learning difficulties", which generally refers to specific learning problems (e.g. dyslexia), rather than a global impairment of intellect and function.

Appendix 22

Risk Factors for Violence in Psychosis

Mullen (1997) very elegantly enumerated the clinical risk factors for violence (towards self or others) among psychiatric patients as follows:
- *Dispositional factors:* Gender, age, marital status, socioeconomic factors, intellectual level, personality and neurobiological factors
- *Historical factors:* Prior history of violence, psychiatric history and personal history
- *Contextual factors:* Current life situation; social support, current emotional state and stress; availability of means; threats of violence or self-harm and substance abuse
- *Illness-related Factors:* The relationship between serious mental illness and violence is very complex, and different recent research generates much debate on this issue (Binder, 1999). Schizophrenia (delusions, hallucinations, passivity experiences and catatonic motor behavior) is most consistently reported to be associated with violent behavior followed by depression (delusions, morbid preoccupations and hopelessness).

The National Institute of Mental Health (NIMH) Clinical Antipsychotic Trials of Intervention Effectiveness (CATIE) project (Swanson et al. 2006) examined the past 6 months violence histories of schizophrenics enrolled in the CATIE treatment trail. "Minor" violence was simple assault without injury or weapon use; "serious" violence corresponded to assault resulting in injury or involving the use of a lethal weapon, threat with a lethal weapon in hand or sexual assault. The 6-month prevalence of any violence was 19%, with 4% of participants reporting serious violence. "Positive" psychotic symptoms, e.g. persecutory delusions, increased the risk of minor and serious violence; negative psychotic symptoms lowered the risk of serious violence. Minor violence was associated with co-occurring substance misuse and interpersonal and social factors. Serious violence was associated with psychotic and depressive symptoms, childhood conduct problems and a history of victimization.

Eronen et al. (1996) in a study of 700 people convicted of homicide in Finland found schizophrenia to increase the risk of homicide (8 fold in men, 6.5 fold in women). Wallace et al. (1998), in a study of individuals convicted of serious offences in Victoria county, Australia, found that those with schizophrenia were more than 4 times more likely to be convicted of interpersonal violence and 10 times more likely to be convicted of homicide than the general population. However, in any given year, only 0.2% of patients with schizophrenia receive a conviction for serious violence. The Epidemiologic Catchment Area (ECA) survey (Swanson et al. 1990), base rate of violence in those without a psychiatric diagnosis is 2%. Schizophrenia or major affective disorder increased the risk to 8%. Addition of substance misuse increased the risk to 30%. Although rates of violence are increased amongst mentally ill, contribution to levels of violence in community, particularly serious violence is quite small.

Delusions: Studies (Taylor, 1985; Mullen et al. 1993) have shown that there is a positive correlation between active delusions and violent behavior. Delusions of persecution and delusions of infidelity (morbid jealousy) are noteworthy in this respect. Taylor (1998) reported that delusions have a definitive role in the precipitation of violent act by people with psychotic illness and there is a correlation between more serious act and more delusions. Any type of delusional symptom whether it is erotomaniac, hypochondriacal or misidentification, has a potential for violent behavior. Dangerous behavior in those with erotomania is more likely if there are multiple delusional objects or there is serious antisocial behavior unrelated to the delusions (Menzies et al. 1995).

Hallucinations: Command hallucinations are regarded as a potentially most dangerous symptom of schizophrenia (Braham et al. 2004). A study (Junginger, 1995) indicates that patients who experience command hallucinations are at risk of dangerous behavior. Some studies found no immediate relation between command hallucinations and violent or suicidal behavior while others indicate a correlation between severity of command hallucination content and compliance (Rudnick, 1999). It is estimated that rates of compliance ranged from 39.2-88.5% and is not consistently related to the dangerousness of commands (Hersh and Borum, 1998). Shawyer et al. 2008 suggested that compliance with harmful commands involves a complex interaction between beliefs related to command, with the risk of compliance with increasing of age and presence of related delusion (Hersh and Borum, 1998).

Passivity experience: Patients who experience their thoughts being controlled by others or thoughts inserted into their head, suffer from loss of self-control and integrity of their own volition and are at risk of responding to fear or rage with violence (Link and Stueve, 1994).

Appendix 23

Interview of Specific Patients and Situations

Not every patient is similar. The psychiatric interview is tailor-made and should be designed according to the special features of each case. There are few distinct situations where the interviewer should orient the interview according to the special demand of the situation, i.e. presenting features of the patient.

■ INTERVIEWING DELUSIONAL PATIENT
- Observe how the patient reacts or defends against painful reactions
- Look for precipitating stress, if any
- Empathically acknowledge the patient's wishes not to be a patient
- Take a natural stance; neither agree with the delusional belief nor openly challenge it
- Focus on other signs and symptoms for which the patient may want help.

■ INTERVIEWING DEPRESSED AND POTENTIALLY SUICIDAL PATIENT
- Not all patients will vocalize their depressive mood freely. They will often provide clues through their verbalizations that indicate a sense of giving up. *Unmasking depression is a skill of the interviewer*
- Look for significant losses and separations in the patient's life
- Take an active role to encourage patient to verbalize what he/she is experiencing
- Enquire about suicidal thought or contemplation; it brings relief to the patient and also helps to arrive at a clinical judgement about the imminent danger of suicide in the patient's life
- Suicidal risk assessment:

Factors	Risks
Sex	Women are more likely to attempt; men are more likely to complete the act
Age	*Bimodal distribution*: Teenagers and the elderly at highest risk
Marital status	Divorced, separated or widowed are at risk
Social	Unemployment, social isolation, low social class

Contd...

Contd...

Factors	Risks
Previous history	History of deliberate self-harm (DSH)*
Depression	15% depressives die by suicide
Past attempt	10% of having history of attempt dies by suicide
Alcohol abuse	15% of alcoholics commit suicide
Loss of rational thinking	Psychosis, 10% chronic schizophrenics die by suicide
Social support	Poor or lacking
Suicidal plan	A well-formulated, organized suicide plan is highly risky
Statement of intent	Two-third of patients who die by suicide have communicated their intent
Family	Family history of suicide (first-degree relatives), recent bereavement
Illness	Chronic illness
Personality	Impulsive personality traits
Means	Easy access to methods (arms, poison, etc.)

Features of high risked past DSH attempt: Attempt planned/attempt done in isolation/precautions taken to avoid rescue/violent method used/Expected fatal outcome/Regrets having been rescued/'Suicide notes' written.

- *Suicidal intent* has been found to be a good predictor of a subsequent suicide attempt. There is a number of risk-predicting score systems to determine suicidal intent, e.g. Beck's Suicidal Intention Scale, Beck's Hopelessness Scale and Inventory of Motivations for Suicide Attempts. The most widely used scales are Pierce Suicide Intent Scale and Beck's Suicidal Intention Scale. These contain about 15 items (scoring from 0–2 points). Part of the scale looks at the patient's thoughts and emotions at the time of the attempt and the other questions are about the circumstances around the attempt.

■ INTERVIEWING PSYCHOSOMATIC PATIENTS

- Patients with psychosomatic illness are usually referred by their primary care physicians and rarely seek psychiatric help from their own. Their greatest fear and anxiety is that the psychiatric consultation is being sought because they are "crazy" or their illness is "mental" or because the referring physician saw no hope for their recovery. This attitude is a part of our social stigma about mental illness.
- Establish your interest in the patient's physical complaints as well as any emotional concomitants.
- Clarify the patient's misunderstanding or apprehension about the psychiatrist's role as professional caregiver skillfully.
- Acknowledge that subjective complaints are real and that your enquiries about emotional concomitants are necessary to gain a better understanding of the patient's distress.

■ INTERVIEWING ELDERLY PATIENTS

- Usually, need to slow the pace of the interview
- Pay special attention to any physical limitations, whether sensory, motor, coordination, extrapyramidal or other

- Need to review the existing medications, both psychotropics and non-psychotropics, carefully
- Show extra courtesy (e.g. assist the patient safely walking in and out of the room or grasping of patient's hands as a signal of reassurance) to the elderly patients.

■ INTERVIEWING VIOLENT/EXCITED PATIENT

- The main issue in approach here is the *safety*, for the patient as well as for the doctor, staff and other persons or patients.
- Make a judgement about the safety of removing physical restraints from the patients.
- Never confront or challenge a violent patient.
- Risk assessment—three aspects: estimate the *seriousness* of the potential harm; estimate the *probability* that the risk will be reality and estimate the *imminence* that the risk will become a reality.
- Practical risk management—vary according to the case and circumstances, but time-scale and urgency are very important. In outpatient department (OPD), try to administer medications to the violent patient as early as possible, so that the agitations could be slowed down reasonably. On inpatient units, use a seclusion room as a temporary placement for violent patients until their behavior is judged not to be dangerous to themselves or to others.

Factors Predicting Violence in Psychiatric Patients (Lipsedge, 2005)

Antecedents	Past history of violence
Diagnosis	Schizophrenia, morbid jealousy or erotomania, substance use, alcohol use
Social/personal factors	Loss of family support, loss of accommodation, relationship breakdown
Clinical	The patient's declared intentions and attitudes to previous and potential victims/threats of violence/presence of active symptoms like delusions, especially about poisoning and sexual matters/passivity experiences/command hallucination/jealousy/depression and angry outburst. Signs and symptoms of relapse of the illness
Management issue	Loss of contact with mental health service/poor compliance with medications

Impulsivity—reflect behavior that is poorly conceived, without previous thought, and is unduly risky or inappropriate to the situation that leads to undesirable consequences.

Aggressively—a verbal or physical attack on other living creatures.

Mental illness may increase the likelihood of committing violence in some patients, but only a small proportion of the violence in society can be ascribed to mental health patients (Mulvey, 1994). Common causes of aggressive behaviors are:
- Comorbid substance abuse, dependence and intoxication
- Symptoms of a psychotic process like delusion or hallucination
- Poor impulse control related to neuropsychiatric deficits

- Personality character like antisocial personality
- Environmental factors like chaotic or unstable home or hospital situation.

INTERVIEWING SEDUCTIVE PATIENT

- Though it is not usual that seductive behavior is apparent in the first interview, yet it is helpful to have some idea of how best to respond to overtly seductive behavior. Always remember the absolute ethical commitment that never to become sexually involved with the patients. Besides breaking of ethical code, such violations are always destructive and damaging to the patient and the physician. Any medical person who often finds himself/ herself tempted to breach this boundary should get therapy or supervision or find another career.
- This does not mean that the practitioner will never have sexual or personal feelings towards their patients. Of course, they will or may have, but if his or her commitment never to act on such feelings is absolute, they can manage these feelings confidently while continuing to deliver appropriate service and care to their clients.
- *Seductive behavior may be expressed in two guises*: (1) subtle and (2) blatant. Subtle behavior includes significant glances, revealing clothes and excessive curiosity about the interviewer's personal life. Blatant seductive behaviors involve more direct questions about the interviewer's availability and requests to be touched or hugged by the therapist or to spend some time with her or him.
- Management of these behaviors needs interviewer's skill and adherence to medical ethics. Psychoanalytic orientation or training is very helpful in this regard.

INTERVIEWING MUTE OR INACCESSIBLE PATIENT

- Mutism is the inability or unwillingness to speak, resulting in the absence or marked paucity of verbal output. It is usually associated with features of an organic or non-organic disorder.
- Stupor is a term used in neurology as a stage on the continuum with comatose, reflecting reduced consciousness. In psychiatry, it usually means a state with preserved awareness with severe psychomotor inhibition. Mutism is always present in stupor.
- Detailed history, physical and full neurological examination.
- Observe whether the patient can articulate or phonate, watch the eye movements (implying an awareness of surroundings) or any purposive movements.
- *Attempt for communication*: Writing or signing. To what extent comprehension affected? Dysphasia due to pure motor Broca's area damage is usually accompanied by frustrated attempts at communication and comprehension is relatively remaining intact.

INTERVIEWING PATIENT WITH ALCOHOL-RELATED PROBLEMS

- Alcohol abuse is a common problem in many psychiatric patients. It may be a cause of, a contributing factor to or a consequence of mental illness.

- It is an important risk factor in suicidal behavior and has serious mental and/or physical consequences.
- Identify the levels of pathology. Three levels: *Excessive drinking* (drinking in excess of safe limits)/*Problem drinking* (excessive drinking with adverse consequences) and *Alcohol dependency* (excessive drinking with physical and psychological dependency).
- History should be addressed to look for signs of chronic alcohol abuse with details of drinking behaviors: What is drunk (nature of drink; beer, spirits or cider)/quantity/money spent on drinks per week/how often per week/where (pub, home or at work)/when (time of the day)/any triggering factor/any period of abstinence/any help sought [Alcoholics Anonymous (AA), counseling or detoxification)/any predisposing factors (family history)].

■ INTERVIEWING A PATIENT WITH POST-TRAUMATIC STRESS DISORDER

- Post-traumatic stress disorder (PTSD) is a psychological and physical condition that is caused by very frightening or distressing events. It occurs in up to 30% of people who experience traumatic events such as military combat, serious road accidents, terrorist attacks, natural or manmade disasters, being held hostage, violent deaths, and violent personal assaults, such as sexual assault, mugging or robbery. PTSD may also occur in any other situation where a person feels extreme fear, horror or helplessness. In some professions PTSD is common like firemen, police, soldiers, working in major disasters.
- PTSD sufferers re-experience the traumatic event or events in some way, tend to avoid places, people, or other things that remind them of the event (*avoidance*), and are exquisitely sensitive to normal life experiences (*hyperarousal*). Delayed PTSD can be triggered by retirement, anniversaries or new similar events.
- PTSD symptoms can range from single symptoms to full-blown illness (flashbacks, panic attacks, emotional numbing, avoidance, nightmares, over-arousal, depression). A secondary psychiatric illness may be a presenting feature.
- A detailed history and genesis of symptoms along with elicitation of time-course with the event are important. PTSD is a medicolegally important disorder because in many instances a possible compensation claim is involved.
- Eliciting the traumatic history may precipitate emotional stress, so utmost care should be taken to unfold the history.

■ INTERVIEWING PATIENT WITH ADULT ATTENTION DEFICIT HYPERACTIVITY DISORDER

- As hyperactivity in various levels is present in attention deficit hyperactivity disorder (ADHD) patients, so long interview may pose difficulty for them to seat long
- As they have difficulties with planning and organizing; so questions and assessment procedure should not be at a rapid pace
- Comorbid mental health problem may pose difficulty in assessment, e.g. anger issue
- Waiting time for ADHD assessment should not be too long otherwise they feel frustrated and impatient.

INTERVIEWING THE PATIENT WITH AN EATING DISORDER

- The interview is very sensitive as the patient tries to hide or deny their eating habits and physical status of health
- The interview should be conducted in a very empathic attitude so that the patient should not perceive the questions as challenging
- The issue of weight phobia and body image disturbances need a very careful clinical probe
- Physical examination to calculate body mass index (BMI) (in anorexia it is 17.5 or less) and menstrual history (amenorrhea; primary or secondary, is essential in the diagnosis of anorexia) should be taken.

INTERVIEWING PERINATAL PATIENT

- Perinatal psychiatry is a very sensitive area in mental health assessment
- The interviewer must have a reasonable degree of empathic and supportive attitude during the assessment
- Emotionality of the patient should be duly addressed
- Informed consent to accept or reject treatment (psychotropic medication during pregnancy) should be thoroughly discussed with evidence-based drug-information materials, and risk-benefits of drug treatment to the mother and the unborn baby should be amply discussed and documented
- It is a good medical practice to discuss the outcome of the assessment with the partner/husband/father of the baby
- A follow-up plan is crucial throughout the gestational period extending to delivery and postpartum.

INTERVIEWING PATIENT FROM ETHNIC MINORITY BACKGROUND

- Understanding cultural factors are very important in the assessment. Perception about their worldview and idioms of distress may help to explain the presenting complaints
- The cultural meaning of symptom experience (like delusion or hallucination) should be carefully delineated in the cultural context
- Immigration history and acculturative stress should be looked for
- Elicitation of Explanatory models of illness (EMI) may help in the treatment negotiation
- In case of questionable linguistic competency, help from the interpreter should be sought for.

INTERVIEWING CHILD AND ADOLESCENT

- Interviewing child and adolescent is a very skilled task and may require a longer time
- Usually, it is not an interview with a single person but multiple individuals, like one of the parents or foster parents or the social worker. Establishment of rapport with all concerned is a hard task

- The usual rule is to interview the child alone, the parent or parents alone and then to talk with everyone together
- Most children are not very much aware of what brings them to the clinic, what the main symptoms are and how long they are suffering
- It is always a good medical practice to obtain a collateral history from the multiple agencies who are working with the child, like pediatrician, therapist, teacher, special education teacher, social worker, counsellor, probation officer, etc. Everyone may contribute valuable information. Releases of information need to be signed
- Diagnosis and treatment plan should be discussed and consented by the parents, guardians and any other involved parties
- Prescribing psychotropic medications, especially for young children, to be conservative.

■ INTERVIEWING RELATIVES

- Please take consent from the patient before interviewing the relatives. Interviewing relatives is very important in psychiatry as it unfolds the patients present functioning, his/her symptom patterns, past history, developmental milestones, social situations as also the family dynamics of the patient; all are essential for a psychiatric understanding of the patient and aid the diagnosis
- Relatives also serve as valuable allies in the treatment process. Their participation is sometimes mandatory for positive treatment compliance
- The relative's participation is contingent on the knowledge and agreement that the psychiatrist cannot, without obtaining consent, divulge to a relative any material that the patient told in confidence to the psychiatrist.

APPENDIX 24

Clinical Risk Management

■ CLINICAL RISK MANAGEMENT

Psychiatric disorders are variously associated with a risk of violence to self or to others. So clinical risk management in mental health service is a very important cornerstone of treatment planning (Lipsedge, 1995).

Clinical Risk Management Steps

1. *Identify and document risk factors*: Formulation of risk for the individual/Weighting of risk(s).
2. *Develop risk management plan*: Based on formulation/Compromise (balance) of risk(s).
3. *Communicate about the plan (in consultation with the consumer/family or caregivers):* May be a written document, face-to-face, consider issues of privacy, crisis management/communication with the team, services, other services, family, other agencies.
4. *Act according to the plan*: In consultation with the consumer, family or caregivers—treatment monitoring, restrictions, environment, use of Mental Health Act.
5. *Evaluation of outcome*: Positive/Negative.
6. *Review the plan in consultation with the consumer, family or caregivers*: A full assessment of any ongoing crisis, identify gaps and consider new inputs.

Some Risk Indicators

Risk to self	*Risk to others*
• Safety (including suicidal acts, deliberate self-harm)	• Violence (including emotional, physical and sexual violence)
• Health (including drug/alcohol abuse; physical or psychological harm)	• Intimidation/threat
• Quality of life (including dignity, social and financial status)	• Neglect/abuse of dependent
• Vulnerability (including exploitation, sexual abuse, violence from others)	• Stalking/harassment
• Self-neglect	• Property damage (including arson)

Contd...

Contd...

Risk to self	Risk to others
• Cultural issues	• Public nuisance
• Spiritual issues	• Reckless behaviors (including driving)
A risk may also be posed to consumers/patients by System or Treatment process itself: side effects of medication; ineffective care; institutionalization; cultural distance and social stigma. These risks are often neglected in management plan but should be carefully considered.	

Positive risk taking is weighing up the potential benefits and harm of exercising one choice of action over another. Identifying the potential risk involved and developing plans and actions that reflect the positive potential and stated priority of the service user.

Balance of risk: In order to achieve a therapeutic gain, it is sometimes necessary to take risks.
- A strategy of total risk avoidance may lead to excessively restrictive management, which may in itself be damaging to the individual.
- Clinical decisions must be based on a thorough and sound analysis of risks and benefits.
- Achievements of beneficial outcome and minimization of harm require a careful judgement of the compromise between various clinical factors.
- The process of balancing risks and benefits must be carefully documented.
- Positive risk-taking should be a collective responsibility.

Cultural risk factors: In assessing and managing risk care should be taken to consider cultural issues:
- Accurate communication
- Different concepts
- Language
- Reluctance to disclose or shame of disclosure
- Family involvement
- Involvement of other healthcare providers—whenever possible, involve someone who is from the patient's culture.

Mental health services should provide staff training in cultural competence and cross-cultural communication issues so that the staff can provide appropriate cultural management.

Standardized Interviews for Suicide Risk Assessment

Rating scale	Suicide risk
Beck Depression Inventory: Patient picks the best answer.	3 = I will kill myself if I had the chance. 2 = I have definite plans about committing suicide. 1 = I feel I would be better off dead. 0 = I do not have any thoughts of harming myself.
Symptom Checklist: Patient rates on a five-point scale from 'not at all' to 'extremely'.	How much were you bothered by: • Thoughts of ending your life? • Thoughts of death or dying?

Contd...

Contd...

Rating scale	Suicide risk
Hamilton Depression Rating Scale: Rater selects the best answer.	0 = Thoughts of suicide absent. 1 = Feels life is not worth living. 2 = Wishes he/she were dead or any thoughts of possible death to self. 3 = Suicide ideas or gesture 4 = Attempts at suicide (any serious attempts rate 4).
Schedule for Affective Disorder and Schizophrenia (SADS): Semi-structured interview. Rater selects answer on a six-point scale from 'not at all' to 'extreme'.	The interviewer asks: When people get upset or feel depressed or feel hopeless, they may think about dying or even killing themselves. Have you? (Have you thought how you would do it? Have you told anybody about suicidal thoughts? Have you actually done anything? Interviewer rates: Suicidal tendencies, including a preoccupation with thoughts of death or suicide. Further questions: Assess gestures, attempts, risk-rescue factors, medical lethality.
Brief Psychiatric Rating Scale: Rater selects answer on a seven-point scale where 1 = Not present and 7 = Extremely severe, on suicidality.	

Appendix 25

Cognitive State Assessment for Organic Brain Disease and Some Neurological Examinations

There is an absolute rule in clinical psychiatry: *The possibility of undisclosed physical disease is part of every differential diagnosis* (Poole & Higgo, 2006). The most common encounter in psychiatry is delirium and dementia.

Delirium: Acute confused state with altered consciousness, impaired awareness of the environment and disturbed cognitive status (attention, orientation and memory) and perceptual disturbances. It runs a fluctuating course with periods of complete or relative lucidity.

Common causes of delirium:
- *Infective*: Non-cerebral (lungs, septicemia), cerebral (meningitis, encephalitis)
- *Brain lesions*: Focal (tumor, cerebrovascular lesions, sub-arachnoid and subdural hemorrhage), diffuse (cerebral hypoxia, raised intracranial pressure)
- Head injury
- *Metabolic*: Electrolyte disturbance, hepatic failure, hypoglycemia
- *Epilepsy*: Post-ictal confusion
- *Drugs*: Intoxication or withdrawal states, especially alcohol
- *Nutritional*: Thiamine deficiency leading to Wernicke's encephalopathy.

Dementia: It is a generalized loss of cognitive abilities without disturbance of consciousness, manifesting in the change of intellect, memory and personality. It is caused by a variety of coarse brain disease, most of which are progressive and irreversible. The commonest causes are Alzheimer's disease, cerebrovascular disease (multi-infarct dementia), Lewy body disease and infectious (HIV, CJD, syphilis).

Mini-Mental State Examination (MMSE, also known as Folstein test—Anthony et al. 1982)

It is a validated, widely used clinical screening tool for cognitive impairment. It is a short and practical instrument that offers a sufficient guide for the cognitive status in the everyday clinical examination.

MMSE Record Form (Folstein, 1975)

Items	Maximum points	Patient score
1. *Orientation:* What is today's day/date/month/season? Where are we? Town/county/country/building/floor?	5 5	
2. *Registration:* Name 3 common objects, e.g. apple, car, ball Ask the patient to repeat all three. Repeat until all three are remembered, number of trials needed:	3	
3. *Attention and concentration:* Start from 100 and keep subtracting 7 Stop after 5 answers (93, 86, 79, 72, 65) OR Spell the word "WORLD" backwards (DLROW)	5	
4. *Recall:* Repeat the three words I asked you to say earlier	3	
5. *Language:* *Naming:* Show a watch and pencil and ask the patient to name them *Repeating:* Repeat the following "no ifs, ands, or buts." *Reading:* Show the sentence "CLOSE YOUR EYES". Read the sentence and do what it says. *Writing:* A short sentence on your own. *Three stage command:* Take a piece of paper in your right hand, fold it in half and place it on the floor.	2 1 1 1 3	
6. *Construction:* Copy the diagram (interlocking pentagons)	1	
TOTAL SCORE	30	

Scoring:

- *Orientation*: 10 points. Ask each question in turn. Probe for a response to each question. Score 1 point for each correct response.
- *Registration*: 3 points. Name three unrelated objects taking about a second for each object. Then ask the patient to repeat all three words. Give one point for each correct answer given at the first attempt. Then repeat all three words until the patient learns all three. If the patient gives an incorrect response after 5 attempts skip item 4.
- *Attention and concentration*: 5 points. Serial 7's. Give one point for each successful subtraction of 7.

OR

Spelling "WORLD" backwards. Deduct one point if a letter is missing or out of sequence (e.g. DLOW 4 points; DRLOW 3 points).

- Recall: 3 points. Score one point for each object recalled.
- Language: 9 points.
  Naming: 2 points. Show a pencil and a watch. Ask the patient to name each in turn.
  Repeating: 1 point. Ask the patient to repeat "no ifs, ands or buts". Score 1 point if successful at first attempt.
  Reading: 1 point. Ask the patient to read and obey the instructions in the sentence "CLOSE YOUR EYES". Score 1 point if the patient closes their eyes.
  Writing: 1 point. Ask the patient to write a sentence. Score 1 point if the sentence contains a subject, verb and object.
  3-Stage command: 3 points. Hand the patient a blank piece of paper and ask to follow the command. Score 1 point for each action completed successfully.
  6. Construction: 1 point. Ask to copy a design. Score 1 point if the shapes have 5 angles and two angles intersect. Ignore size, tremors and rotation of pentagon.

The Mini-Cog Test: It is a 3-minute instrument used to detect cognitive impairment in older adults. It consists of three steps: (1) Three Word Registration/(2) Clock drawing/(3) Three Word Recall. As a screening test, however, it does not substitute for a complete diagnostic workup. (Available at www.alz.org/documents_custom/minicog.pdf).

Six-item Cognitive Impairment Test (6CIT): It is a simple dementia screening tool. Cognition assessment toolkit is a very important clinical help provided by Alzheimer Society and Department of Health, UK, which is available at https://www.alzheimers.org.uk/download/downloads/id/3475/alzheimers_society_cognitive_assessment_toolkit.pdf.

Parietal Lobe Disorders

Patients with left parietal lobe lesions have receptive aphasia and thus unable to understand questions. Right parietal lobe lesions cause problems in sustaining and directing attention. Moreover, parietal lobe disorder patients may be either unaware of their defects or unable to communicate with the examiner, so collateral history is very important. During MSE, careful attention should be given to locating—language problems, problems with distribution of attention, visual, spatial or constructional defect, body image distortions, tactile or motility disturbances.

Parietal Lobe Tests

Dominant parietal lobe tests	
Finger agnosia:	Ask the patient to name which finger you touched. Touch two fingers on each side
Left-right disorientation:	Ask the patient to put his/her right hand on the table, then remove it. Repeat with the left hand, then right hand again
Praxis:	Ask the patient to mime how he/she combs hair, use scissors, clean teeth, blow out a match. Watch for inability to do these and also for the use of body parts as objects (cleans teeth with a finger)
Calculation:	Ask the patient to write down five numbers and add them up

Contd...

Contd...

Writing:	Ask the patient to write a sentence
Overlapping pentagons test (in MMSE)	Test for constructional dyspraxia—tests for dominant parietal lobe sign
Non-dominant parietal lobe tests	
Postural arm drift:	Ask the patient to hold out the arms, palms down, eyes closed. Watch for drift of either hand downwards. Arm drift indicates contralateral parietal lobe abnormality
Unilateral neglect:	Ask the patient, eyes closed, to tell you which hand you touched. Touch left, right, both together

Frontal Lobe Syndrome

It is caused by frontal lobe damage, tumor or infarction. There is a lack of judgement, a coarsening of personality, disinhibition, pressure of speech, lack of planning ability, and sometimes apathy. Perseveration and a return of the grasp reflex may occur.

Assessment of Frontal Lobe Functioning

Dubois et al. (1994) suggested that the skills necessary for the elaboration, control and execution of goal-directed behaviors form the basis of testing the activity of the prefrontal cortex. These abilities include planning, mental flexibility, impulse control, working memory and evaluation of one's behavior—that is the executive process.

Common Tests to Assess Executive Functions (Goldman et al. 2004):

Function	Tests
Abstract thinking	Comprehension subset of Wechsler adult intelligence scale—revised/Gorham's proverbs test (Common proverbs are read, and the subject is asked to indicate the general meaning)
Concept formation, social judgment	Similarities subsets of Wechsler adult intelligence scale-revised
Concept formation and cognitive flexibility including establishing, maintaining and shifting cognitive set	Wisconsin card sorting test/Halstead categories test
Cognitive flexibility and psychomotor speed	Trail making test—part B
Cognitive set maintenance and impulse control	Stroop color-word test
Planning and impulse control	*Porteus* Maze test
Visual-spatial working memory and problem solving	Tower of London test
Cognitive productivity	Controlled Oral Word Association test (verbal fluency)/Ruff figure fluency test (design fluency)

Clinical Bedside Frontal Lobe Tests (Poole and Higgo, 2006)

Grasp reflex	Test by stroking both the patient's palms. An abnormal response is a reflex grasp of the stroking fingers
Motor sequencing	Ask the patient to watch what you do and copy. Then, with arms outstretched, palms down, alternate opening and closing fists (as one fist opens the other closes). Alternatively Luria test—tap on the desk in a repeating sequence of closed fist on the desk, the edge of open hand on the desk, palm down on the desk. Repeat fist, edge, palm several times and ask the patient to copy.
Perseveration	Ask the patient to tap three times on the table with his/her middle finger.
Alternating frames of reference	Ask the patient to tap once on the table when you tap once. Then to tap twice when you tap twice. Then to tap twice when you tap once. Then to tap once when you tap twice.

Paresis is a condition of partial loss of movement or impaired movement. Usually, paresis means weakness, and plegia to describe paralysis in which all movement is lost. Clinical features help to differentiate between paresis of central origin from peripheral paresis (Mumenthaler & Mattle, 2004).

Clinical feature	*Central paresis*	*Peripheral paresis*
Proprioceptive muscle reflexes	Increased	Decreased
Exteroceptive muscle reflexes	Decreased	Decreased
Babinski sign	Present	Absent
Muscle atrophy	Absent or mild	Present
Muscle tone	Increased	Decreased

Different types of paresis: Monoparesis: One leg or one arm/Hemiparesis: One arm and one leg on either side of the body/Paraparesis: Both legs or both arms/Quadriparesis: All four limbs.

Lesions and Clinical Picture of Hemiparesis

Site of lesion	*Clinical picture*
Cerebrum	Spastic hemiparesis, may involve facial muscles, characterize by ↑ muscle tone, ↑ reflexes, pyramidal tract signs, no atrophy, usually with a sensory deficit
Brainstem	Spastic hemiparesis as above, face involvement depends on the level of lesion, cranial nerve deficits contralateral to hemiparesis
Upper cervical spinal cord	Spastic hemiparesis as above, face spared, possible ipsilateral loss of position and vibration sense and contralateral loss of pain and temperature sense below the level of the lesion (Brown-Sequard syndrome)

Lesions and Clinical Picture of Para or Quadriparesis

Site of lesion	*Clinical picture*
Cerebrum (bilateral lesion)	Clinical picture of "bilateral hemiparesis" or paraparesis due to a bilateral parasagittal cortical lesion
Corticobulbar pathways in the brainstem (bilateral lesion)	Bilateral spasticity with mild weakness, spastic, small-stepped gait, hyperreflexia, pyramidal tract signs, no sensory deficit, usually with pseudobulbar signs (dysarthria, hyperreflexia of the facial musculature)
Corticospinal pathways in the spinal cord (bilateral lesion)	Para or quadri, face spared, hyperreflexia, pyramidal tract signs, no sensory deficit, mild weakness

Clinical Features of Increased Intracranial Tension:

Subjective	Headache—diffuse and persistent, most severe in the morning, vomiting (fasting, projectile), apathy
Signs of impending herniation	Confusion, respiratory difficulties, bradycardia, hypertension, cerebellar fits (opisthotonus and extensor spasms of arms and legs), dilated pupil
Ocular signs	Papilledema, enlarged blind spots, attacks of amblyopia, oculomotor palsy, occasional abducens palsy
Skull X-ray	Increased digitate markings, enlarged sella turcica with demineralized dorsum sellae
CT/MRI	Slit ventricles, periventricular signal change, possible lesion tumor or hemorrhage
EEG	Diffuse abnormal, nonspecific
LP	Contraindicated

Clinical Features of Brain Tumors:

Signs/symptoms	Objective findings
Headache—early symptom in one third	Focal neurological deficits
Intracranial hypertension	Vomiting, bradycardia may not always present, neuropsychological and psychopathological abnormalities
Epileptic seizures	Initial symptom in one fourth
Neuropsychological changes	Apathy, irritability, memory impairment, papilledema common

General Differential Diagnosis of Brain Tumors:

Space-occupying lesion other than a tumor	Chronic subdural hematoma, brain abscess, arachnoid cyst
Encephalitis:	Herpes encephalitis, brainstem encephalitis, multiple sclerosis
Vascular pathology:	Stroke in progress, intracerebral hemorrhage, arteriovenous malformations, giant aneurysm

- *Extrapyramidal syndromes:* The extrapyramidal system (caudate nucleus, putamen, globus pallidus, subthalamic nucleus, substantia nigra and red nucleus on both sides) is involved in motor functions. Disorders may produce either an abnormal decrease of muscle tone (hypotonia) or an abnormal increase in tone (rigidity). So these may result in either an overall paucity of movement (hypokinesia) or superfluous movements like tremor, chorea, athetosis and other involuntary movements. Common extrapyramidal syndromes include:

Syndrome	Clinical features
Parkinsonism	Akinesia, rigidity, resting tremor
Progressive supranuclear palsy (Steele-Richardson-Olszewski disease)	Downward gaze palsy, rigidity, pyramidal signs, retraction of the head, subcortical dementia
Chorea	Irregular, rapid, asymmetric, mainly distal involuntary movements
Athetosis	Irregular, slow, mainly distal involuntary movements at varying sites, with joint hyperflexion and hyperextension

Contd...

Contd...

Syndrome	Clinical features
(Hemi)-ballism	Irregular, sudden, large amplitude, ballistic involuntary movement of an entire limb or limbs
Dystonic syndromes: • Spasmodic torticollis • Torsion dystonia • Localized dystonias	Involuntary tonic contractions of shorter or longer duration affecting individual muscles or muscle groups (against the resistance of antagonist muscles)
Hepatolenticular degeneration (Wilson's disease)	Progressive "wing-beating" tremor, rigidity, dysarthria, mental changes, hepatic dysfunction, corneal Kayser-Fleischer ring
Myoclonus	Involuntary, irregular, rapid, brief twitches of individual muscles or muscle groups

- *Electroencephalogram (EEG):* It involves recording the spontaneous electrical activity of the brain using surface electrodes applied to the scalp. The electrodes are attached at standardized positions, and the small electrical signals that are detected are amplified, displayed and recorded. An 8 or 16-channel tracing is usually used when the patient is awake or asleep. The signals can be modified or enhanced by active hyperventilation, sleep deprivation or photic stimulation.

Normal EEG Wave Forms (Malhi et al. 2000)

Rhythm	Frequency (Hz)	Features
Alpha	8–13	Symmetrical, parieto-occipital region, enhanced by eye closure, disappears with eye-opening
Beta	>13	Symmetrical, frontal. Unaffected by eye-opening
Theta	4–8	Frontal and temporal predominance. Occurs normally during sleep, abnormal during wakefulness
Delta	<4	Frontal and temporal predominance. Occurs normally during sleep, abnormal during wakefulness

Pathologic EEG Rhythms and their Clinical Significance

EEG waves	Clinical significance
Focal slow activity	Localized cerebral lesion, e.g. infarct, hemorrhage, tumor, abscess, encephalitis
Intermittent, rhythmic slow waves	Thalamocortical dysfunction, metabolic or toxic disturbances, obstructive hydrocephalus, posterior fossa lesion, nonspecific findings in generalized epilepsy
Generalized arrhythmic and polymorphic slow activity	Diffuse encephalopathy of metabolic, toxic, infectious or degenerative origin
Epileptiform discharges: focal or generalized spikes, sharp waves, or spike-slow wave complexes	Focal or generalized epilepsy
Low-voltage activity	Hypoxic-ischemic brain injury, degenerative brain diseases, subdural hematoma

Contd...

Contd...

EEG waves	Clinical significance
3 Hz bilateral, symmetrical spike-and-wave activity	Typical absence seizure
Generalized multiple spike-and-wave activity	Myoclonic epilepsy
Flat-line	Consistent with but not diagnostic of brain death

Tardive Dyskinesia

Tardive dyskinesia (TD) is a mostly irreversible disorder of involuntary movements caused by long-term use of antipsychotic drugs (chlorpromazine HCl, thioridazine HCl, haloperidol, perphenazine, thiothixene, trifluoperazine HCl, and fluphenazine HCl). About 20% of people taking antipsychotics for more than one year become affected by TD. The prevalence of TD tends to be highest among elderly patients and among women.

The symptoms include tongue protrusion, grimacing, rapid eye blinking, lip smacking, pursing, or puckering, rapid movement of the arms or legs and other involuntary movements of the head, face, neck and tongue muscles. There is no standard treatment for TD. The primary approach is to discontinue or minimize the use of antipsychotic drugs or replace it by second-generation antipsychotics (atypical).

Neurological Causes of Hallucination

Perception of the external world depends on a very complex physiological process. The stimuli received through eyes and ears processed in the brain at many levels to form a meaningful mental image. The process starts in the brainstem, pass to the limbic system and finally involve the temporal, parietal and occipital areas of the cerebral cortex. Various types of hallucination are caused by disruptions that occur at different levels along that sequence of this brain processes.

- *Damage to the upper brainstem*—produces *peduncular hallucinations* of faces, torsos and occasionally geometric patterns or landscapes near the viewer at the close of day. The images may be static, vivid, chromatic or may change in content and affective tonality while being viewed. Usually, the hallucinatory experience is multimodal—they are seen, heard, and even touched, and occur over the entire visual field. Olfactory and gustatory images have also been described. Peduncular hallucinations are similar to the hypnagogic hallucinations that are experienced when falling asleep.
- *Damage of limbic and temporal lobe structures* yields hallucinations of faces or formed scenes laden with meaning and affect. Changes in size (micropsia, macropsia) and shape (metamorphopsia) may occur. Déjà vu, derealization, and dreamy states are common. Auditory hallucinations are usually of speech or music. Microscopic (Lilliputian) and autoscopic (out-of-the-body) hallucinations also occur with temporal-lobe lesions.
- *Damage to the parietal lobe* leads to illusory distortions of shape, size, and motion, whereas occipital lesions or stimulation—or migraine—gives elementary hallucinations of sparks,

flames, lines, or simple patterns. These hallucinations share features with afterimages. *Palinopsia* is the hallucinatory persistence of an object after the viewer has turned away, is a form of pathological afterimagery.

Symptom triad: Positive-Negative-Cognitive Symptoms in Schizophrenia

Clinically the signs and symptoms of schizophrenia may be divided into three categories: positive, negative and cognitive symptoms as follows:

Positive symptoms	Negative symptoms	Cognitive symptoms
That are *added* to the personality, i.e. symptoms that are 'extra' due to additional brain activity, reflects a loss of touch with reality	Reflects under-functioning or 'loss' of personality—loss of emotional range and interpersonal function	Cognitive dysfunction involving multiple areas of brain functioning
Delusions: Bizarre delusions are considered characteristic of schizophrenia. Delusions of persecution are most common	*Affective flattening*: A diminished range of emotional expression, flat or blunted affect, poor eye contact, reduced body language	*Difficulty maintaining attention:* Difficulty in getting and remaining focused on any task or even a thought; not being able to pay attention to instructions or directions
Hallucinations: These may occur in all the sensory modalities, but auditory hallucinations are most common	*Alogia*: Decreased fluency and productivity of speech—poverty of speech, such as brief, empty replies	*Memory problems*: Difficulties with normal 'working memory', which involves the capacity to use information immediately after it has been presented and/or learned
Thought disorder: Difficult speaking and organizing thoughts, 'formal thought disorder' is considered typical for schizophrenia	*Avolition*: Lack of motivation, inability to initiate and persist in goal-directed activities, show little interest in participating in work or social activities	*Low executive functioning*: Problem with understanding information and acting upon that to make decisions
Disorganized behavior: Difficulties in goal-directed behavior or odd and inappropriate behavior	*Anhedonia:* Inability to experience pleasure in things that they once found enjoyable	*Difficulty planning and structuring activities:* Caused by reduced executive control
Catatonic motor behavior: Any type: extreme degree of complete unawareness (catatonic stupor) or maintaining a rigid posture and resisting efforts to be moved (catatonic negativism) or the assumption of inappropriate or bizarre postures (catatonic posturing), or purposeless and unstimulated excessive motor activity (catatonic excitement)	*Asociality*: Lack of desire to form relationships	*Lack of insight*: Caused by loss of reality testing, having a specific cognitive blind spot that prevents them from understanding that they are ill and need treatment

APPENDIX 26

Grief, Bereavement and Complicated Grief

Grief is a natural response to losing someone or something that's important to the person.

Five common stages of grief are: Denial; Anger; Bargaining; Depression and acceptance.

For conceptual clarity of different terms used in this context, Zisook and Shear (2009) define the commonly used terms as follows:

- Bereavement refers to the fact of the loss; the term grief should then be used to describe the emotional, cognitive, functional and behavioral responses to the death.
- Mourning (sometimes used interchangeably with bereavement and grief), refers to the behavioral manifestations of grief, which are influenced by social and cultural rituals, like funerals, visitations, or other customs like personal or community expression of mourning.
- *Complicated grief, also* referred to as unresolved or traumatic grief, is a syndrome of prolonged and intense grief that is associated with substantial impairment in work, health, and adaptive social functioning.

Persistent complex bereavement disorder (PCBD): For a subset of people, feelings of loss are debilitating and do not improve even with the passing of time. This is known as *complicated grief*, also called *persistent complex bereavement disorder (PCBD)*. In complicated grief, painful emotions are so long lasting and severe that the individuals never fully integrate the loss into their life and continue to experience severe disruption in daily life many years after the loss event (Arizmendi & O'Connor, 2015). Complicated grief lasts longer than 6 months.

Differential Diagnosis of Persistent Complex Bereavement Disorder

Normal grief: Persistent complex bereavement disorder usually lasts longer, and severely interfering with the sufferer's functioning long after the death.

Depressive disorder: PCBD shares features like sadness with major or persistent depressive disorder, but this depressed mood is characterized by a focus on the loss only.

Post-traumatic stress disorder: Individuals with post-traumatic stress disorder may suffer intrusive thoughts about a traumatic event, while in PCBD they may suffer thoughts about the deceased or the circumstances of their death.

Separation anxiety disorder: Separation anxiety disorder applies to separation from a living individual, whereas sufferers of PCBD people experience anxiety when separated from the deceased.

Complications of PCBD: Complicated grief can affect the person physically, mentally and socially. Without appropriate treatment, complications may include: Depression; Suicidal thoughts or behaviors; Anxiety, including PTSD; Significant sleep disturbances; Increased risk of physical illness (e.g. heart disease, cancer or high blood pressure); Long-term difficulty with daily living, relationships or work activities and Alcohol, nicotine use or substance misuse.

Bereavement exclusion in DSM-5: Persistent complex bereavement disorder is included in the DSM-5 chapter that outlines areas for further study. DSM-5 removed the "bereavement exclusion" from both depression and adjustment disorders: that a person who is grieving a loss potentially may be diagnosed with depression or an adjustment disorder. It is the removal of the bereavement exclusion from these diagnoses and has generated lots of debate.

Reasons for exclusion (Pies, 2012): (1) "There have never been any adequately-controlled, clinical studies showing that major depressive symptoms following bereavement differ in nature, course, or outcome from depression of equal severity in any other context—or from MDD appearing "out of the blue"; and (2) Major depression is a potentially lethal disorder, with an overall suicide rate of about 4%. Disqualifying a patient from a diagnosis of major depression simply because the clinical picture emerges after the death of a loved one risks closing the door on potentially life-saving treatment".

Appendix 27

Diagnostic and Statistical Manual of Mental Disorders (DSM-5)

The Diagnostic and Statistical Manual of Mental Disorders (DSM-5) was published by American Psychiatric Association on May 18, 2013, superseding the DSM-IV-TR. DSM-5 for the first time using Arabic numeral instead of a Roman numeral.

DSM-IV TR or Diagnostic and Statistical Manual, text revision was published in June 2000. The previous editions were: DSM-I in 1952, DSM-II in 1968, DSM-III in 1980, DSM-IIIR in 1987 and DSM-IV in 1994.

The DSM-5 has four sections:
- *Section 1*: It includes an introduction and instructions on how to use the new version.
- *Section 2*: It covers the diagnostic categories (22 in total).
- *Section 3*: Emerging measures and models—assessment measures; Cultural formulation; Alternative DSM-5 model for personality disorders and conditions for further study.
- *Section 4*: Appendix that includes glossary of technical terms, glossary of cultural concepts of distress; Alphabetical/numerical listing of DSM-5 diagnoses and codes.

Some salient changes in DSM-5 (Lane, 2013):
- *No more multiaxial assessment system:* DSM-5 has discarded the multiaxial system of diagnosis (formerly Axis I, Axis II, Axis III), listing all disorders in Section II. It has replaced Axis IV with significant psychosocial and contextual features and dropped Axis V (Global Assessment of Functioning, known as GAF). The World Health Organization's (WHO) Disability Assessment Schedule is added to Section III (Emerging measures and models) under Assessment Measures, as a suggested, but not required, method to assess functioning.
- *Restructured order of chapters*: The order of chapters (22 in all) with related disorders/chapters grouped together, e.g. one of the new chapters is Trauma- and Stressor-Related Disorders", which will include PTSD.
- *New diagnoses*:
  – Disruptive mood dysregulation disorder
  – Hoarding disorder
  – Binge Eating disorder
  – Excoriation disorder

- *Revised diagnoses*:
  - Autism Spectrum Disorder
  - Posttraumatic Stress Disorder
  - Pedophilic Disorder
  - Substance Use Disorder
  - Specific Learning Disorder
  - Removal of Bereavement Exclusion
- *Disorders requiring further research:* The DSM-5 includes Attenuated Psychosis Syndrome (a precursor to schizophrenia), Internet Use Gaming Disorder, Non-Suicidal Self-Injury, and Suicidal Behavioral Disorder in this section. It is important to note that they still need more research.

History of DSM:
- First DSM: DSM-I in 1952
- Second DSM: DSM-II in 1968
- Third DSM: DSM-III in 1980; DSM-IIIR in 1987
- Fourth DSM: DSM- IV in 1994; DSM IV TR (Text-Revised) in 2000
- Fifth DSM: DSM-5 in 2013.
  [Highlights of changes from DSM-IV- TR to DSM by APS (2013) is available at APA website]

APPENDIX 28

International Classification of Diseases, 10th Revision, WHO (1992)

WHO incorporated a section on mental disorders in the sixth edition of ICD in 1952. The latest edition is the 10th edition, published in 1992. Chapter V (F) is reserved for mental and behavioral disorders. Each mental disorder section contains a brief glossary notes about the content of the categories. For the easy applicability by the mental health staff, ICD has several specific versions for different purposes, e.g. clinical descriptions and diagnostic guidelines CDDG version for clinical psychiatrists; diagnostic criteria for research DCR version for research workers in the field of psychiatry; multiaxial version for classification of mental disorders which allows simultaneous assessment of different aspects of the patient's illness (e.g. levels of impairment and disability, change overtime, environment etc.); primary health care PHC version for general or primary care practitioners and the ICD-10 PA (psychiatric and neurological adaptations) for easy use in psychiatry-neurology related health services.

Each of the categories of ICD-10 has a code composed of 4 characters. First of all, there is a letter designating the chapter usually a group of diseases of particular interest to a medical specialty. The second numerical digit describes a subgroup of disorders, e.g. affective disorders. The third character, also a digit, describes the disease or disorder and the fourth character, a digit, gives more detail about the condition, e.g. describing its form or course.

F20.10
- F: Mental disorder chapter
- 2: Section of schizophrenia and related disorders
- 0: Schizophrenia
- 1: Type of schizophrenia = hebephrenia
- 0: Type of course = continuous.

ICD-10 Categories

ICD codes	Disorders
F00 – 09	Organic, including symptomatic mental disorders
F10 – 19	Mental and behavioral disorders due to psychoactive substance use
F20 – 29	Schizophrenia, schizotypal and delusion disorders

Contd...

Contd...

ICD codes	Disorders
F30 - 39	Mood (affective) disorders
F40 - 48	Neurotic, stress related and somatoform disorders
F50 - 59	Behavioral syndromes associated with physiological disturbances and physical factors
F60 - 69	Disorder of adult personality and behavior
F70 - 79	Mental retardation
F80- - 89	Disorder of psychological development
F90 - 98	Behavioral and emotional disorders with onset during childhood and adolescence

ICD Multiaxial Classification

ICD Axis I   Corresponds to DSM-IV, Axis I, II and III combined.

ICD Axis II   Deals with the disability due to an impairment produced by the illness from which the individual suffers. Ratings are made on a 5-point scale for four areas of functioning. This corresponds to DSM-IV, Axis V.

ICD Axis III Is for recording environmental factors and personal life factors which influence the course and outcome of the disease. This corresponds to DSM-IV, Axis IV.

ICD-10 Diagnostic Criteria for Major Mental Illness*

Dementia	Delirium

• Disease of the brain
• Chronic or progressive nature
• Disturbance of multiple higher cortical functions including:
  – Memory
  – Thinking
  – Orientation
  – Comprehension
  – Calculation
  – Learning capacity
  – Language
  – Judgement
  – Consciousness is not clouded.
	• Organic cerebral syndrome
	• Disturbances of:
	  – Consciousness
	  – Attention
	  – Perception
	  – Thinking
	  – Memory
	  – Psychomotor behavior
	  – Emotion
	  – Sleep-wake schedule
	  – Severity ranges from mild to very severe

Schizophrenia	
Positive symptoms	Negative symptoms
• Thought echo; thought insertion or withdrawal; thought broadcasting • Delusions • Delusional perception • Delusions of control; influence or passivity • Hallucinatory voices (discussing the patient) • Overvalued ideas • Catatonic behavior • Breaks or interpolations in the train of thought • Persistent hallucinations occurring in any modality (everyday for weeks or months)	• Blunted affect • Apathy loss of drive (avolition) • Social isolation • Poverty of speech • Poor self-care

Contd...

Contd...

Mania	Depression
• Symptoms/features for 7 days with sustained dysfunction: 　– Elevated mood 　– Distractible 　– Poor concentration 　– Flight of ideas 　– Pressure of speech 　– Increased energy 　– Expansive grandiose ideas 　– Disinhibited behavior 　– Decreased need for sleep *Hypomania,* as the name suggests, has to be present for 4 days with only mild/moderate dysfunction, insight tends to preserve.	• Symptoms for 2 weeks with sustained dysfunction: 　– Lowering of mood 　– Anhedonia 　– Reduction of energy 　– Decreased concentration 　– Reduced self-esteem and self-confidence 　– Ideas of guilt or worthlessness 　– Somatic symptoms 　– Psychomotor retardation 　– Poor sleep 　– Early morning waking 　– Worse in morning 　– Loss of appetite 　– Loss of weight 　– Loss of libido

Panic disorder (episodic paroxysmal anxiety)	Generalized anxiety disorder
• Recurrent attacks of severe anxiety (panic). • Somatic symptoms • Feelings of unreality depersonalization or derealization. • Recurrent over 1 month	• Anxiety that is generalized and persistent • Complaints of persistent nervousness, trembling, muscular tensions, sweating, lightheadedness, palpitations, dizziness, and epigastric discomfort • May fluctuate

Obsessive-compulsive disorder	Phobic anxiety disorder
• Recurrent obsessional thoughts or compulsive acts • Obsessional thoughts are ideas, images, or impulses that enter the patient's mind, involuntary and often repugnant • Compulsive acts or rituals are stereotyped behaviors that are repeated to prevent some objectively unlikely event, often involving harm to or caused by the patient • Anxiety worsens if compulsive acts are resisted	• Anxiety certain well-defined situations (not at present dangerous) • Situations avoided or endured with dread (anticipatory anxiety) • Symptoms like palpitations or feeling faint • Secondary fears of dying, losing control, or going mad • Phobic anxiety and depression often coexist

Substance misuse	
Harmful use	**Dependence syndrome**
• Psychoactive substance use that is causing damage to health • Can be physical (e.g. hepatitis) or mental (e.g. episodes of depressive disorder secondary to heavy consumption of alcohol). *Withdrawal state:* • Variable group of symptoms • Occurring withdrawal of a psychoactive substance after persistent use • Related to the type of substance and dose used immediately before cessation • State may be complicated by convulsions	• Behavioral, cognitive, physiological phenomena develop after repeated substance use which can include: • Strong desire to take the drug • Difficulties in controlling its use • Persisting in its use despite harmful consequences • A higher priority given to drug use than to other activities and obligations • Increased tolerance • Sometimes a physical withdrawal state

*WHO International Classification of Diseases (ICD) http://www.who.int/classifications/icd/en/.
*The work on ICD-11 is ongoing and expected to be published soon. The updates are available at ICD-11 website.

Appendix 29

Personality Disorders

Diagnosis in DSM-5 and ICD-10 both recognize that patient has a personality trait that interacts and often contributes to the development of a psychiatric disorder. It is very difficult to diagnose a personality disorder in the first interview, yet careful delineation of the life history of the patient during history taking and symptom clue form the complaints may help to develop an insight about any coexisting personality disorder. Carlat (1999) provided a very useful way to examine the presence of personality disorder symptoms by noting the following behavioral clues with an expected number of symptoms to be present for the probable diagnosis.

■ CARLAT'S (1999) FLOWCHART

1. *Eccentric Cluster:* Paranoid, Schizoid, Schizotypal

Paranoid: Patient appears guarded and suspicious; answers questions reluctantly with an air of suspicion	*Schizoid:* Patient appears shy and aloof, seems to be preoccupied in his/her own kingdom	*Schizotypal:* Patient appears odd like disheveled, wearing strange clothes or have odd mannerisms, describes strange ideas, bordering psychotic dimension
Mnemonic: **SUSPECT (4 of the 7):** S = Spousal infidelity suspected U = Unforgiving S = Suspicious of others P = Perceives attacks E = Enemy or friend C = Confiding in others feared T = Threats perceived in non-threat or simple events	Mnemonic: **DISTANT (4 of the 7):** D = Detached or flattened affect I = Indifferent to criticism or praise S = Sexual experience—little interest T = Tasks or activities performed solitarily A = Absence of close friends N = Neither desires nor enjoys close relations T = Takes pleasure in few activities	Mnemonic: **ME PECULIAR (5 of the 10):** M = Magical thinking or odd beliefs E = Experiences unusual perceptions P = Paranoid ideation E = Eccentric behavior or appearance C = Constricted or inappropriate affect U = Unusual (odd) thinking and speech L = Lack close friends I = Ideas of reference A = Anxiety in social situations R = Rule out psychotic disorder and pervasive developmental disorder

2. Dramatic Cluster: Borderline, Antisocial, Histrionic, Narcissistic

Borderline: Alternatively idealize and devalue the examiner during the interview, emotionally labile.

Mnemonic: **I DESPAIR**
I = Identity disturbance
D = Disordered, unstable affect owing to a marked reactivity of mood
E = Emptiness feelings, chronic
S = Suicidal behavior/gestures, threat, mutilating behavior—recurrent
P = Paranoid ideation, transient or stress-related
A = Abandonment, frantic effort to avoid real or imagined abandonment
I = Impulsivity
R = Rage, inappropriate or difficulty controlling anger

Antisocial: The patient is excessively cocky and arrogant, portrays self as innocent and a victim in violent or criminal circumstances.

Mnemonic: **CORRUPT (3 of the 7)**
C = Conformity to law lacking
O = Obligations ignored
R = Reckless disregard for the safety of self or others
R = Remorse lacking
U = Underhanded—deceitful, lies
P = Planning insufficient or impulsive
T = Temper

Histrionic: The patient is flamboyantly and seductively groomed or dressed, is dramatically self-revealing

Mnemonic: **PRAISE ME (5 of the 8):**
P = Provocative (or seductive) behavior
R = Relationships (considered more intimate than they are)
A = Attention—uncomfortable when not the center of attention or attention-seeking behavior
I = Influenced easily (suggestibility)
S = Style of speech—impressionistic, lack-detail often vague
E = Emotions—rapidly shifting and shallow
M = Make-up for the occasion; physical appearance used to draw attention
E = Exaggerated emotions (theatrical)

Narcissistic: The patient is of complaining type, excessively critical of others and has much resentment about how unfairly others have treated him/her

Mnemonic: **SPEEECIAL (5 of the 9):**
S = Special—believes he/she is special and unique
P = Preoccupied with fantasies (about success or power)
E = Envious
E = Entitlement
E = Excessive admiration required
C = Conceited
I = Interpersonal exploitation
A = Arrogant
L = Lacks empathy

3. Anxious Cluster: Avoidant, Dependent, Obsessive-compulsive

Avoidant: The patient may appear shy and nervous but eager to make contact in the course of the interview, may open up and self-revealing

Mnemonic: **CRASIEN (4 of the 7):**
C = Certainty of being liked required before willing to risk involvement
R = Rejection—possibility preoccupies thoughts
A = Avoid intimate relationships
S = Self-viewed as unappealing, inferior

Dependent: The patient will seem to make extraordinary attempts to gain the examiner's affection

Mnemonic: **RELIANCE (5 of the 8):**
R = Reassurance (required for decisions)
E = Expressing disagreement difficult (fear of loss of support or approval)
L = Life responsibilities assumed by others

Obsessive-compulsive: The patient is meticulously groomed and dressed, give an excessively detailed and accurate account of symptoms

Mnemonic: **LAW FIRMS (4 of the 8):**
L = Loses point of activity
A = Ability to complete tasks compromised by perfectionism
W = Worthless objects (unable to discard)
F = Friendships (and leisure activities) excluded

Contd...

Contd...

I = Inter-personal contact avoidance in occupational activities E = Embarrassment potential prevents new activities N = New relationships avoided	I = Initiating projects difficult A = Alone (feels helpless) N = Nurturance (try excessively to obtain nurturance and support) C = Companionship sought urgently when a close relationship ends E = Exaggerated fears of being left to care for self	I = Inflexible, over conscientious R = Reluctant to delegate M = Miserly S = Stubborn

In DSM-5, the ten different personality disorders can be grouped into three clusters based on descriptive similarities within each cluster. These clusters are:

1. *Cluster A (the "odd, eccentric" cluster):* It includes paranoid personality disorder, schizoid personality disorder, and schizotypal personality disorders. The common features of the personality disorders in this cluster are social awkwardness and social withdrawal. These disorders are *dominated by distorted thinking*.
2. *Cluster B (the "dramatic, emotional, erratic" cluster):* It includes borderline personality disorder, narcissistic personality disorder, histrionic personality disorder and antisocial personality disorder. Disorders in this cluster share problems with impulse control and emotional regulation.
3. *Cluster C (the "anxious, fearful" cluster):* It includes avoidant, dependent, and obsessive-compulsive personality disorders. These three personality disorders share a high level of anxiety.

ICD-10 Classification of Personality Disorders*

F60.0	Paranoid personality disorder
F60.1	Schizoid personality disorder
F60.2	Dissocial personality disorder
F60.3	Emotionally unstable personality disorder
F60.4	Histrionic personality disorder
F60.5	Anankastic personality disorder
F60.6	Anxious (avoidant) personality disorder
F60.7	Dependent personality disorder
F60.8	Other specific personality disorder
F60.9	Personality disorder unspecified
F61	Mixed and other personality disorders
F62	Enduring personality changes , not attributable to brain damage and disease
F62.0	Enduring personality changes after catastrophic experience
F62.1	Enduring personality changes after psychiatric illness
F62.8	Other enduring personality changes
F62.9	Enduring personality changes, unspecified

* http://apps.who.int/classifications/icd10/browse/2016/en#/F68

Appendix 29: Personality Disorders | **157**

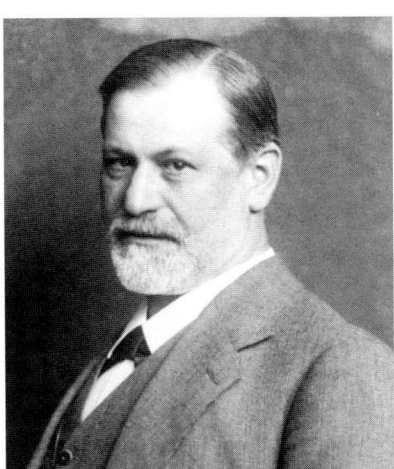

Sigmund Freud (6.5.1856 – 23.9.1939), an Austrian neurologist, psychiatrist and father of Psychoanalysis. He unfolded the operational structure and function of the mind.

Appendix 30

Ego Defense Mechanisms

Sigmund Freud (1920) postulated a trivalent topographical theory of mind which is as follows:
- *Conscious mind* is what we are aware of at any particular moment, our present perceptions, memories, thoughts, fantasies and feelings.
- Working closely with the conscious mind is the *preconscious mind*, may be called "available memory"—anything that can easily be made conscious, the memories we are not at the moment thinking about but can readily bring to mind if needed. It has access to both conscious and unconscious mind. It uses secondary process thinking.
- The third part is the *unconscious mind* which includes all the things that are not easily available to awareness including the drives or instincts, and things that are put there because we do not want to face them like traumatic memories and emotions. The unconscious is the source of all motivations, whether they are simple desires for food or sex, neurotic compulsions, or the motives of an artist or scientist. It uses primary process thinking.

In his psychoanalytic theory, Freud in 1923 postulated that the personality is composed of three elements (structural theory) known as id, ego and superego work together to guide and create human behaviors.

Id: It is the only component of personality that is present from birth and is the source of all psychic energy, making it the primary component of personality.
- Id is entirely unconscious.
- Contains all the instinctive drives and responsible for our primitive behaviors.
- Ruled by the *pleasure principle*, which strives for immediate gratification of all desires, wants, and needs. If these needs are not satisfied immediately, the result is a state of anxiety or tension.
- No awareness of reality.

Ego: It is responsible for dealing with reality. The ego develops from the id and ensures that the impulses of the id can be expressed in a manner acceptable in the real world. The ego functions in the conscious, preconscious and unconscious mind.
- Second structure to develop.
- Operates on reality principle.
- Mediates conflict among id, ego and superego.
- Provides reality testing.

- Monitors quality of interpersonal relations.
- Provides synthesis and coordination.
- Defends against anxiety.

The ego operates on the basis of the reality *principle* which strives to satisfy the id's desires in realistic and socially appropriate ways. In many cases, the id's impulses can be satisfied through a process of delayed gratification—the ego will eventually allow the behavior, but only in the appropriate time and place. The ego also discharges tension created by unmet impulses through the *secondary process* in which the ego tries to find an object in the real world that matches the mental image created by the id's primary process.

Superego: The last component of personality to develop and holds all of our internalized moral standards and ideals that we acquire from both parents and society—our sense of right and wrong, just or unjust.
- Self-criticism based on moral values.
- Self-punishment.
- Self-praise based on ego-ideal
- Most functions are unconscious.

According to Freud, the superego begins to emerge at around age five. There are two parts of the superego: (a) *Ego ideal* which includes the rules and standards for good or acceptable behaviors. Obeying these rules leads to feelings of pride, value and accomplishment. (b) The *Conscience* which includes information about things that are viewed as bad by parents and society. These behaviors are often forbidden and lead to bad consequences, punishments or feelings of guilt and remorse.

Primary and secondary processes: In the ego, there are two ongoing processes. First, there is the *unconscious primary process*, where the thoughts are not organized in a coherent way, the feelings can shift, contradictions are not in conflict or are just not perceived that way, and condensations arise. There is no logic and no timeline. Lust is important for this process. By contrast, there is the *conscious secondary process*, where strong boundaries are set, and thoughts must be organized in a coherent way.

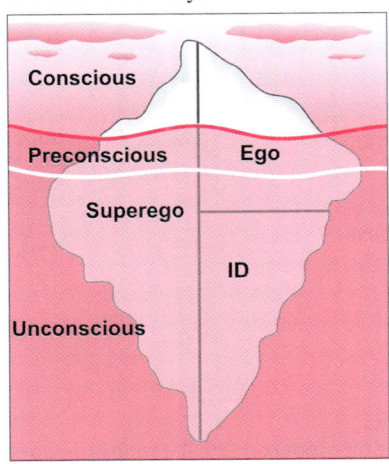

The iceberg metaphor is often used to explain the psyche's parts in relation to one another.(http://www.simplypsychology.pwp.blueyonder.co.uk/freud-personality.html)

The Interaction of the Id, Ego and Superego

With so many competing forces, both instinctual and external, it is easy to see how the conflict might arise between the id, ego and superego. Freud used the term *ego strength* to refer to the ego's ability to function despite these dueling forces. A person with good ego strength is able to effectively manage these pressures, while those with too much or too little ego strength can become too unyielding or too disrupting. In fact, the key to a healthy personality is a balance between id, ego, and superego.

In Freud's topographical model of personality, the ego is the aspect of personality that deals with reality. While doing this, the ego also has to cope with the conflicting demands of the id and superego. Id seeks to fulfill all wants, needs and impulses, while superego tries to get the ego to act in an idealistic and moral manner. What happens when the ego cannot deal with the demands of our desires, the constraints of reality and our own moral standards? This situation generates *anxiety*—an unpleasant inner state that people seek to avoid. Anxiety acts as a signal to the ego that things are not going right. Freud identified three types of anxiety:

1. *Reality anxiety*: This is the most basic form of anxiety and is typically based on fears of real and possible events. The most common way of reducing tension from reality anxiety is taking oneself away from the situation.
2. *Neurotic anxiety*: This anxiety comes from an unconscious fear that the basic impulses of the Id will take control of the person leading to eventual punishment.
3. *Moral anxiety*: This anxiety comes from the superego in the form of a fear of violating values, moral codes and appears as feelings of guilt or shame.

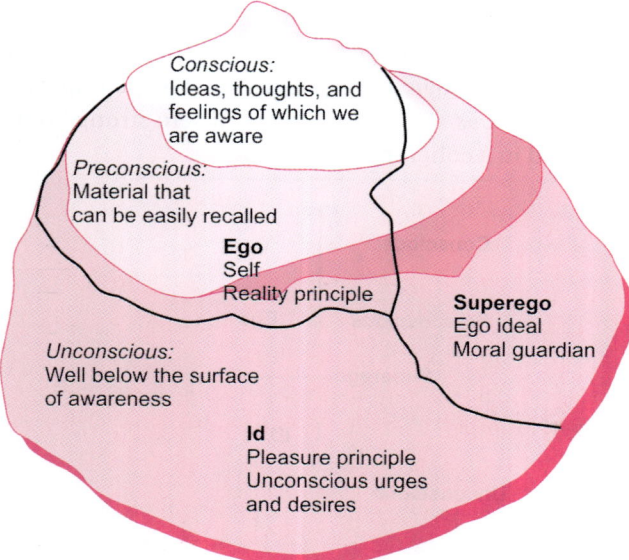

Id-Ego-Superego interactions
(http://jamielzillseniorport.blogspot.com/2010/11/idea-id-ego-super-ego.html)

Defense Mechanisms

The ego deals with the demands of reality, id, and superego as best as it can. But when the anxiety becomes overwhelming, the ego must defend itself. It does so by unconsciously blocking the impulses or distorting them into a more acceptable, less threatening form. The techniques are called *ego defense mechanisms*. These are tactics which the ego develops to help deal with Id and SuperEgo. All defense mechanisms share two common properties—(a) they often appear unconsciously, and (b) they tend to distort, transform, or otherwise falsify reality. In distorting reality, there is a change in perception which allows for a lessening of anxiety with a corresponding reduction in felt tension.

The list of defense mechanisms is huge, and there is no theoretical consensus on the number of defense mechanisms. Different theorists have different categorizations and conceptualizations of defense mechanisms. Following is a brief classification (Vaillant, 1977) to be useful in clinical psychiatry:

Pathological defenses: Often called Narcissistic or psychotic defenses. Persistent use of these defenses may lead to maladaptive behavior that will eventually threaten the physical and/or mental health of the individual. These are common in overt psychosis, in dreams, and throughout childhood.

Delusional projection: Grossly frank delusions about external reality, usually of a persecutory nature.

Denial: Refusal to accept or acknowledge a painful or threatening external reality. Many people use denial in their everyday lives to avoid dealing with painful feelings or areas of their life they do not wish to admit, e.g. a person who is a chronic alcoholic will often simply deny they have a drinking problem, pointing to how well they function in their job and relationships.

Distortion: A gross reshaping of external reality to meet internal needs.

Splitting: A primitive defense. Negative and positive impulses are split off and unintegrated. Divides external objects into 'all good' and 'all bad'. It is a tendency to make gross good-bad distinctions, e.g. the belief that all left politicians are bad, all persons of a specific ethnic group or particular community are inferior and selfish.

Immature defenses: Often present in adults and more commonly in adolescents. These defenses lessen distress and anxiety provoked by threatening people or situations. People who excessively use such defenses are seen as socially undesirable in that they are immature, difficult to deal with and seriously out of touch with reality. These defenses are often seen in severe depression and personality disorders. In adolescence, the occurrence of all of these defenses is normal.

Acting out: Direct expression of an unconscious wish or impulse in action, without conscious awareness of the emotion that drives that expressive behavior, e.g. a child's temper tantrum is a form of acting out when he/she does not get his/her way with a parent. Self-harm is a form of acting out, expressing in physical pain what one cannot stand to feel emotionally.

Fantasy: Tendency to retreat into fantasy in order to resolve inner and outer conflicts.

Idealization: Overestimation of the desirable qualities and underestimation of the limitations of a desired object, e.g. a lover speaks in glowing terms of the beauty and intelligence of an average looking woman who is not very bright.

Passive aggression: Aggression towards others expressed indirectly or passively, such as using procrastination. It is a personality trait marked by a pervasive pattern of negative attitudes and passive, usually disavowed resistance in interpersonal or occupational situations.

Projection: Projection is a primitive form of paranoia. Projection also reduces anxiety by allowing the expression of the undesirable impulses or desires without becoming consciously aware of them; attributing one's own unacknowledged, unacceptable/unwanted thoughts and emotions to another, e.g. an angry spouse accuses their partner of hostility. This defense mechanism is commonly overutilized by paranoid persons.

Projective identification: Placing unwanted aspects into another person so that the projector feels at one with an object, e.g. a person who doubts his/her own intelligence level and attempts to manipulate other perceptions/opinions by discourse with "elevated airs" or by referring to themselves as having a high IQ or implied superior knowledge/expertise.

Turning against the self: Inappropriate feeling towards others is redirected to oneself, e.g. attempt to use self-harm to deal with anger towards others. An important mechanism in the psychodynamics of suicide.

Somatization: Conflicts are represented by physical symptoms involving parts of the body innervated by the sympathetic and parasympathetic system, e.g. a highly competitive and aggressive person whose life situation requires that such behavior is restricted, develops hypertension.

C. Neurotic defenses: Such defenses have short-term advantages in coping, but can often cause long-term problems in relationships, work and in enjoying life when used as one's primary style of coping with the reality.

Displacement: Redirecting emotions to a substitute target, e.g. being angry at the boss and kicking the dog.

Dissociation: Temporary drastic modification of one's personal identity or character to avoid emotional distress; separation or postponement of a feeling that normally would accompany a situation or thought (e.g. fugue states, hysterical conversion, identity disorder). A person who dissociates often loses track of time or themselves and their usual thought processes and memories. People who have a history of childhood abuse often suffer from some form of dissociation. In extreme cases, dissociation can lead to a person believing they have multiple selves (multiple personality disorder).

Hypochondriasis: An excessive preoccupation or worry about having a serious illness.

Intellectualization: A form of isolation; concentrating on the intellectual components of a situation so as to distance oneself from the associated anxiety-provoking emotions, e.g.

an individual who when told they had a life-threatening disease focuses exclusively on the statistical percentages of recovery and is unable to cope with their fear and sadness.

Isolation: The splitting-off of the emotional components from a thought, e.g. a bank cashier appears calm and cool while frustrating a robbery but afterward is tearful and tremulous. The mechanism of isolation is commonly overutilized by OCD patients.

Rationalization (making excuses): Offers rational explanations to justify attitudes, beliefs, behaviors instinctually based. Rationalization is often called the "sour grapes defense" (Aesop's fables), e.g. a woman with dozens of shoes buys a new pair because she does not have anything to wear.

Reaction formation: Expression of exaggerated ideas and emotions that are the opposite of one's repressed beliefs or feelings, e.g. a young mother who is furious at her child and wishes her harm might become overly concerned and protective of the child's health.

Regression: Temporary reversion of the ego to an earlier stage of development rather than handling unacceptable impulses in a more adult way, e.g. an adolescent who is overwhelmed with fear, anger and growing sexual impulses might become clinging and begin thumb sucking or bedwetting.

Repression: Unconsciously expelling the anxiety-provoking ideas or feeling from conscious awareness, e.g. a traumatized soldier has no recollection of the details of a terrific bloody encounter with death.

Undoing: It is the attempt to take back behavior or thoughts that are unacceptable. A person tries to 'undo' an unhealthy, destructive or otherwise threatening thought by engaging in the contrary behavior, e.g. excessively praising someone after having insulted them.

D. Mature defenses: Commonly found among emotionally healthy adults. The use of these defenses enhances pleasure and feelings of control and helps to integrate conflicting emotions and thoughts.

Altruism: Constructive service to others that brings pleasure and personal satisfaction, e.g. after the death of wife, the person keeps himself busy by volunteering at the church.

Anticipation: Realistic planning for future discomfort.

Asceticism: The elimination of directly pleasurable affects attributable to an experience. Uses morals to assign values to specific pleasures. Derives gratification from renunciation of all consciously-perceived base pleasures.

Humor: Overexpression of unpleasant or threatening ideas and feelings that gives pleasure to others, e.g. a person's treatment for cancer makes him lose his hair, so he makes jokes about being bald.

Identification: The unconscious modeling of one's self upon another person's character and behavior, e.g. a young doctor without being aware that he is copying his teacher, assumes a similar mode of dress and manner with patients.

Introjection: Identifying with some idea or object so deeply that it becomes a part of that person, e.g. when a person becomes depressed due to the loss of a loved one, his feelings are directed to the mental image he possesses of the loved one.

Sublimation: The conversion and channeling of unacceptable emotions into socially condoned behavior. It is a healthy redirection of an emotion, e.g. a woman is forced to undertake a restrictive diet; she becomes interested in painting and does a number of still life pictures, most of which include fruit or intense rage redirected in the form of participation in sports, such as boxing or football.

Suppression: The conscious or semiconscious decision to postpone attention to a conscious impulse or conflict. At times, suppression may lead to subsequent repression, e.g. a young man at work finds that he is letting thoughts about a meeting with his fiancé that evening interfere with his duties; he decides not to think about plans for the evening until he leaves work.

Individuals use several types and instances of ego defenses mechanisms in their daily lives. These are merely ways in which they respond to anxieties, impulses or threats that arise from the id-demand. Defense mechanisms are triggered by fears, desires, emotional conflicts and perceived threats or stress. Some defense mechanisms (e.g. projection, splitting, and acting out) are almost invariably maladaptive. Others, such as suppression and denial, may be either maladaptive or adaptive depending on their severity, their inflexibility, and the context in which they occur. So the question is: When is a defense mechanism considered really "adaptive" and when is it considered "pathological"? These are the issues that make a defense "pathological":

- The defense is used in a rigid, inflexible, and exclusive manner.
- The motivation for using the defense comes more from past needs than present or future reality.
- The defense severely distorts the present situation
- Use of the defense leads to significant problems in relationships, functioning, and enjoyment of life.
- Use of the defense impedes or distorts emotions and feelings, instead of rechanneling them effectively.

Freudian psychologists consider ego defense mechanisms as natural responses to various forms of anxiety. Defense responses are not coping mechanisms. Coping mechanisms are characterized as conscious and rational, whereas defense mechanisms are irrational and subliminal.

[More examples are available at www.coldbacon.com/**defense**s.html, www.planetpsych.com/...101/defense_mechanisms.html].

Some Pioneers of Psychoanalytical Psychiatry

Carl Gustav Jung (1875-1961), was a Swiss psychiatrist and psychotherapist who founded "analytical psychology". His work has a deep impact not only in psychiatry but also in philosophy, anthropology, archaeology, literature, and religious studies. The central concept of analytical psychology is *individuation*—the psychological process of differentiation of the self out of each individual's conscious and unconscious elements. He introduced the concept "Collective unconscious" to represent a form of the unconscious common to mankind as a whole and originating in the inherited structure of the brain.

Alfred W Adler (1870-1937), was an Austrian medical doctor, psychotherapist, and founder of the school of "individual psychology". His emphasis was on the importance of feelings of inferiority—the inferiority complex— which plays a key role in personality development.

Hermann Rorschach (1884-1922), was a Swiss Freudian psychiatrist and psychoanalyst, best known for developing a projective test known as the *Rorschach inkblot test*. This test was designed to reflect unconscious parts of the personality that "project" onto the stimuli. In the test, individuals are shown 10 inkblots—one at a time—and asked to report what objects or figures they see in each of them.

Melanie Reizes Klein (1882-1960), was an Austrian-British psychoanalyst who devised novel therapeutic techniques for children. She was a leading innovator in theorizing *object relations* theory.

Helene Deutsch (1884-1982), a Polish-American psychoanalyst, was one of the most prominent female leaders in psychoanalysis. She was the first woman to lead Sigmund Freud's Vienna Psychoanalytic Society, and she contributed significantly to a theory on the psychology of women that expanded the purview of Freud's male dominant ideas about women.

Karen Horney (1885-1952), was a German psychoanalyst. Her theories questioned some traditional Freudian views. This was particularly true of her theories of sexuality and of the 'instinct orientation' of psychoanalysis. She is credited with founding feminist psychology in response to Freud's theory of penis envy. She disagreed with Freud about inherent differences in the psychology of men and women, and she put stress on society and culture rather than biology.

Franz Gabriel Alexander (1891-1964), was a Hungarian-American psychoanalyst and physician, who is considered one of the founders of psychosomatic medicine, because of his leading role in identifying emotional tension as a significant cause of physical illness and psychoanalytic criminology.

Michael Balint (1896-1970), was a Hungarian psychoanalyst. He was a proponent of the Object Relations school. He introduced the concept of the "basic fault" that illness is the result of early environmental factors which result in helplessness. He founded the "Balint Groups" in which physician-members discuss the care of patients and the doctor-patient relationship.

Margaret Schönberger Mahler (1897-1985), was a Hungarian physician, interested in psychiatry. She was a prominent figure in the world stage of psychoanalysis. Her main interest was in normal childhood development and developed the *"separation-individuation"* theory of child development.

Anna Freud (1895-1982), the youngest child of Sigmund Freud, was a founder of child psychoanalysis. Anna Freud is known as well for *"The Ego and the Mechanisms of Defense* (1937)", in which she emphasized the role of the ego as the seat of observation, discussed the various defense mechanisms and elaborated on the concept of defense in relation to reality.

Girindrasekhar Bose (1887-1953) was an early 20th century South Asian medical doctor and psychoanalyst from Kolkata, India, the first president (1922-1953) of the Indian Psychoanalytic Society. He founded the Indian Psychoanalytical Society in Kolkata in 1922. Bose carried on a twenty year dialogue with Sigmund Freud. Known for disputing the specifics of Freud's Oedipal theory, he was probably an early example of non-Western contestations of Western methodologies. He developed an eastern notion of "repression" (1921)—by blending of Hindu thought and Freudian concepts.

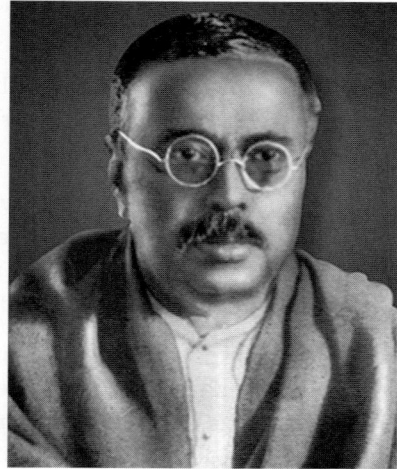

Girindrasekhar Bose (30.1.1887–3.6.1953)

Appendix 31: Some Pioneers of Psychoanalytical Psychiatry

Erik Homburger Erikson (1902–1994), was a German-born American developmental psychologist and psychoanalyst known for his theory on psychosocial development, comprising of eight stages from infancy to adulthood. During each stage, the person experiences a psychosocial crisis which could have a positive or negative outcome for personality development. He was famous for coining the phrase "identity crisis".

John Bowlby (1907–1990), was a psychoanalyst and believed that mental health and behavioral problems could be attributed to early childhood. He created the evolutionary theory of *attachment,* which suggests that children come into the world biologically pre-programmed to form attachments with others because this will help them to survive.

Appendix 32

Psychiatric Report

Written reports on patients are often asked from different judicial or nonjudicial agencies. Usual requests fall into one of the four broad groups:

1. *Purpose*:
   - Protection of the public or institutions (life assurance and mortgage companies, licensing authorities—fitness to drive, employment agencies—fitness to work, occupational physicians—sick leave)
   - Protection of the patient from judiciary—competence, fitness to plead, civil contracts etc. Mental Health Act—inpatient care, treatment provision)
   - Child Protection (about the child's mental illness or of the parents)
   - Medico-legal and Compensation proceedings (nature of psychiatric disorders and prognosis)
2. *Guiding rules:*
   - *Confidentiality*: Written consent must be obtained from the patient before dispatching personal information to an outside agency. In some situations like where the duty of care to the public or to a child overrides the duty of confidentiality and in such situation the psychiatrist may write the report even without the patient's consent.
   - *Impartiality*: The report is from an expert professional and must not be biased in favor of one side or another. It should not be influenced by the interest of the commissioning agency, and the report should be written with the best interest of the patient.
   - *Clarity*: Language and the focus of the report should be simple and goal-directed, avoiding as much possible the use of technical terms, if used, should be defined and explained.
3. *Consent:*

Consent for the release of medical information to a third party must be obtained prior to a medico-legal report being prepared. The following criteria must be met for consent to be valid:
   - The subject (or their legal guardian) must be competent to provide it;
   - It must be informed. That is, the subject must have a clear understanding of the implications of the release of the information;

- It must be specific;
- It must be freely given. A release of privileged medical information in a medico-legal report without valid consent is unethical and may be illegal.

4. Structure:
   - *Part one*: Details of you, your designation and in what capacity writing this report, when and where.
   - *Part two*: Details of patient's identifying data and the reference of commissioning agency.
   - *Part three*: List the sources of information/interview used for this report.
   - Part four: Patients detail clinical data including background, diagnosis, treatment prognosis and recommendations.
   - *Part five*: Answering the specific questions/purpose for which the report is asked.
   - *Part six*: Statement of truth and your signature with date.

[A statement of truth is a statement signed by you to verify that the contents of the report are true. The usual format of Statement of Truth runs like this:
- I understand that my duty is to the Courts, both in preparing reports and in giving oral evidence. I have set out in my report what I understand from those instructing me to be the questions in respect of which my opinion as an expert is required.
- I confirm that insofar as the facts stated in my report are within my own knowledge. I have made clear which they are, and I believe them to be true and that the opinions I have expressed represent my true and complete professional opinion.
- I will notify those instructing me if for any reason I subsequently consider that the report requires any correction or qualification.]

Appendix 33

Commonly Used Rating Scales in Psychiatry

A. *Psychiatric Screening Tests:*
   - *SRQ-20*: Self Reporting Questionnaire (WHO)
   - *GHQ-28*: General Health Questionnaire
   - *PSI-2*: Psychological Screening Inventory

B. *Diagnostic Scales:*
   - *CIDI*: Composite International Diagnostic Interview
   - *PSE-9*: Present State Examination, 9th Edition
   - *PRIME-MD*: Primary Care Evaluation of Mental Disorders
   - *SADS*: Schedule for Affective Disorders and Schizophrenia
   - *SCAN*: Schedule for Clinical Assessment in Neuropsychiatry
   - *SCID*: Structured Clinical Interview for DSM-IV Axis I Disorders

C. *General Anxiety:*
   - *HAM-A*: Hamilton Rating Scale for Anxiety
   - *STAI*: State-Trait Anxiety Inventory

D. *Phobia/Social Anxiety:*
   - *FQ*: Fear Questionnaire
   - *SPAI*: Social Phobia and Anxiety Inventory

E. *Panic Disorder:* API: Acute Panic Inventory

F. *OCD: Y-BOCS-* Yale-Brown Obsessive-Compulsive Scale

G. *CAPS:* Clinician-Administered *Post-Traumatic Stress Disorder*: PTSD Scale

H. *Depression:*
   - *BDI*: Beck Depression Inventory
   - *HRSD*: Hamilton Rating Scale for Depression
   - *MADRAS*: Montogomery-Asberg Depression Rating Scale

I. *Bipolar Disorder:*
   - *YMRS*: Young Mania Rating Scale
   - *MDQ*: Mood Disorders Questionnaire

J. **Psychosis:**
   - *BPRS*: Brief Psychiatric Rating Scale
   - *CPRS*: Comprehensive Psychopathological Rating Scale
   - *PANSS*: Positive and Negative Symptom Scale for Schizophrenia
   - *SANS*: Scale for Assessment of Negative Symptoms
   - *SAPS*: Scale for Assessment of Positive Symptoms
K. **Assessment of Functional Level:**
   - *CGI*: Clinical Global Impressions
   - *GAF*: Global Assessment of Functioning
L. **Personality Tests:**
   - *MMPI*: Minnesota Multiphasic Personality Inventory—personality and emotional status
   - 16PF questionnaire
   - *Projective tests*: TAT, Rorschach Inkblots.
M. **Personality Disorder:**
   - *SHI*: Self-Harm Inventory
   - *MMPI-BPD*: Minnesota Multiphasic Personality Inventory- Borderline Personality Disorder
   - *PDQ-4*: Personality Diagnostic Questionnaire-4
   - *MCMI*: Millon Clinical Multiaxial Inventory.
N. **Adult ADHD:**
   - Adult ADHD Self-Report Scale (ASRS-v1.1) Symptom Checklist
   - Diagnostic Interview for ADHD in adults (DIVA)
   - Wender Utah Rating Scale for the Attention Deficit Hyperactivity Disorder.
O. **Risk Assessments:**
   - *PCL-R*: Hare Psychopathy Checklist-Revised
   - HCR-20, Version 2: Historical, Clinical, Risk
   - Pierce Suicide Intent Scale (to be completed after a suicide attempt).
P. **Side Effects Scale:**
   - *AIMS*: Abnormal Involuntary Movement Scale
   - *SAS*: Simpson-Angus Scale
   - *ESRS*: Extrapyramidal Symptom Rating Scale.
Q. **Addiction:**
   - *ASI*: Addiction Severity Index
   - CAGE Questionnaire (screening test for Alcohol Dependence).
R. **Others:**
   - *DAI*: Drug Attitude Inventory. Patient's attitude towards treatment.
   - *WHOQOL*: WHO Quality of Life
   - *BSS*: Beck Scale for Suicide Ideation
   - *SRRS*: Social Readjustment Rating Scale
   - Medical Outcomes Study Short Form (SF 36: Health status scale).

S. *Dementia:*
   - Neuropsychiatric Inventory (NPI)
   - Clinical Dementia Rating (CDR)
   - Disability Assessment for Dementia (DAD).
T. *Neuropsychologic Tests:*
   - Halstead-Reitan Battery for cognitive and adaptive ability including language and memory.
   - Luria-Nebraska Neuropsychological Battery for brain-damaged patients.
   - Wechsler Adult Intelligence Scale for clinical assessment of intelligence for patients between 16-74 years age. *Two components*: Verbal scale (information, digit span, vocabulary, arithmetic, comprehension, similarities) and performance scale (picture completion, picture arrangement, block designs, object assembly, digit symbol).
   - Stanford-Binet, 4th Edition—Test for age-graded general intelligence.
   - *Raven's progressive matrices*: A test of visuospatial analysis, spatial conceptualization and numerical reasoning.
   - *Bender Gestalt Test*: A test for constructional ability. Screening for organicity/ brain damage.
U. *VAS and CGI-I:*

   Two scales are frequently used in regular clinical practice. They are simple and easy to use.
   1. *Visual Analog Scale (VAS):* It is a simple measurement instrument that measures a characteristic or attitude that is believed to range across a continuum of values and cannot easily be directly measured. It is often used in epidemiologic and clinical research to measure the intensity or frequency of various symptoms. VAS can be presented in a number of ways, including:
   - Scales with a middle point, graduations or numbers (numerical rating scales)
   - Meter-shaped scales (curvilinear analogue scales)
   - "Box-scales" consisting of circles equidistant from each other (one of which the subject has to mark), and
   - Scales with descriptive terms at intervals along a line (graphic rating scales or Likert scales).
   - In its simplest form, VAS is a straight horizontal line of fixed length usually 100 mm. The ends are defined as the extreme limits of the parameter to be measured (symptom, pain, health) orientated from the left (worst) to the right (best). For example, the pain VAS is a unidimensional measure of pain intensity:

   Numeric pain scale (NPS) for pain severity measurement

0	1	2	3	4	5	6	7	8	9	10
No pain										Most pain

   VAS can be tailored made according to the purpose, for example, measuring the intensity of mood or delusional conviction or improvement of symptoms overtime (serial VAS).

2. *Clinical Global Impression-Improvement Scale (CGI-I):* It is a 7-point scale that requires the clinician to assess how much the patient's illness has improved or worsened relative to a baseline state at the beginning of the intervention. The usual ratings are:
   1. Very much improved
   2. Much improved
   3. Minimally improved
   4. No change
   5. Minimally worse
   6. Much worse
   7. Very much worse

Clinical Global Impression (CGI) also used as an efficacy index for measures of symptom severity, treatment response and the efficacy of treatments in treatment studies of patients with mental disorders (Guy, 2000).

Appendix 34

Commonly Used Laboratory Tests in Psychiatry

During care-planning and treatment negotiation both clinical indication, efficacy and side effects of the prescribed medicine should be thoroughly discussed with the service user, if needed he/she may be provided with written information. Many of the psychotropic medication has serious side effect profile and need baseline and periodic blood tests and monitoring.

Atypical antipsychotics, particularly clozapine and olanzapine, have serious side effect profiles clinically known as 'Metabolic syndrome'. Metabolic syndrome refers to a complex medical condition associated with abdominal obesity; abnormalities in glucose, lipid, and cholesterol metabolism; and elevated blood pressure that increases the risk of cardiovascular disease (CVD) and type 2 diabetes. Baseline and periodic testing for glucose, liver function test (LFT), lipid profile are mandatory.

Hematologic side effects of psychotropic medications (e.g. agranulocytosis, neutropenia, eosinophilia, thrombocytopenia, leukocytosis, impaired platelet aggregation, and anemia) need periodic complete blood count (CBC). Some typical and atypical antipsychotic (especially risperidone and amisulpride) cause symptomatic hyperprolactinemia. Symptoms of hyperprolactinemia include amenorrhea, galactorrhea, infertility, loss of libido and erectile dysfunction. Resulting hypogonadism may cause osteoporosis.

Therapeutic drug monitoring: The rationale behind therapeutic drug monitoring is that drug metabolism varies from patient to patient and that the plasma level of a drug is more closely related to the drug's therapeutic effect or toxicity than is the dosage. For example, drugs with a narrow therapeutic index (where therapeutic drug levels do not differ greatly from levels associated with serious toxicity) should be monitored like lithium, phenytoin, digoxin. Therapeutic drug monitoring involves not only measuring drug concentrations, but also the clinical interpretation of the result which requires knowledge of the pharmacokinetics, sampling time, drug history and the patient's clinical condition. It can also be used to detect toxicity, so therapeutic drug monitoring can optimize patient management and improve clinical outcomes (Ghiculescu, 2008).

Serum lithium estimation at regular interval is a part of lithium (Li) treatment protocol. Baseline and periodic cardiac, thyroid and kidney functioning assessment is essential for those who are on Lithium (Li).

The standard blood collection time for a lithium level measurement is 12 hours postdose after a person has been receiving the same dosage for at least a week.

The desired serum level of lithium (Severus et al. 2008) is:
- For mania, mixed mania, and maintenance in bipolar disorder, the therapeutic range is 0.6–1.2 mEq/L.
- Levels below 0.6 render significantly less protection from a manic relapse.
- In acute mania, it is sometimes necessary to increase the level to 1.5 mEq/L, although at the cost of increased adverse effects.
- For maintenance treatment in a reasonably stable person with bipolar I disorder, a generally acceptable serum level is 0.6–0.75 mEq/L.
- Lithium toxicity can occur in the therapeutic range but becomes more significant at levels of 2 mEq/L and higher. At higher serum levels, the risk of renal disease and the need for dialysis increase.
- In the event of acute toxicity (>2 mmol/L) lithium should be stopped immediately and hemodialysis may be started to reduce the blood lithium level. Factors increasing toxicity are: Renal impairment, sodium depletion, diuretic therapy, old age.

Clozapine is associated with neutropenia (incidence 3%) and agranulocytosis (0.8%), so clozapine monitoring is mandatory. Full blood count to be done weekly for first 18 weeks, fortnightly until 52 weeks of treatment and then monthly thereafter if hematological profile remains stable (Taylor et al. 2007).

For serum clozapine level:
- The standard blood collection time for clozapine levels should be 12 hours postdose because its half-life is 12 hours.
- Laboratory report for a serum clozapine level includes the levels of clozapine and its primary metabolites, N-desmethylclozapine (norclozapine)
- The current recommendation is to make clinical decisions based solely on the serum clozapine level (Freudenreich, 2009).
- Clozapine levels in the range of 100–250 ng/mL tend to be less effective than higher levels, but they may be adequate in some patients.
- Clozapine levels in the range of 250–350 ng/mL are commonly associated with a good clinical response.
- If a patient has not responded after an adequate period with a level between 250 and 350 ng/mL, it is reasonable to increase the clozapine dosage to achieve a 12 hours postdose serum clozapine level between 350 and 500 ng/mL.
- Clozapine levels greater than 1,000 ng/mL should be avoided because there is a significant increase in adverse effects including seizures.
- Cigarette smoke and caffeine intake are potent inducer of CYP1A2 which are the primary metabolic pathway for clozapine; thus, these can result in a 50% reduction in the serum clozapine level (Dratcu et al. 2007).

■ COMMON TESTS

Complete blood count: Hematocrit/Hemoglobin/White Blood Cell Count (WBC)/WBC differential/Red Blood Cell Count (RBC)/RBC Indices/, Mean Corpuscular Volume (MCV), Mean Corpuscular Hemoglobin (MCH), Mean Corpuscular Hemoglobin Concentration (MCHC)/stained red cell examination (peripheral smear)/platelet count

Liver function test (LFT): Albumin/globulin (A/G) ratio/albumin/alkaline phosphatase/aspartate aminotransferase (AST)/bilirubin (total, direct (conjugated), indirect (unconjugated)/hepatitis B surface antigen/serum gamma-glutamyl transferase (SGGT)/serum glutamic-oxaloacetic transaminase (SGOT)/ serum glutamic-pyruvic transaminase (SGPT)/lactate dehydrogenase (LDH)/prothrombin time

Kidney function test: A/G ratio/albumin/blood urea nitrogen (BUN)/creatinine/creatinine clearance/globulins/LDH/phosphorus/total protein/urine analysis/uric acid

Lipid profile: Cholesterol [total, low-density lipoprotein (LDL), high-density lipoprotein (HDL), very low-density lipoprotein (VLDL))/triglycerides]

Thyroid function test: Triiodothyronine (T3)/thyroxine (T4)/Free T4/T7 (free thyroxine index, FTI), thyroid stimulating hormone (TSH)

Electrolytes: Calcium/chloride/phosphorus/magnesium/potassium/sodium

Glucose: Oral glucose tolerance test is ideal. Random plasma glucose or glycosylated hemoglobin (HbA1c) in both fasting is not required, may be useful.

Folic acid: Folic acid is required for the synthesis of DNA and the normal functioning of RBCs and WBCs. Its deficiency cause anemia. Decreased levels of folic acid are often seen in malnutrition, liver disease associated with alcoholism, pregnancy, megaloblastic anemia, hemolytic anemia, hyperthyroidism, some cancers, drugs (alcohol, anticonvulsants, antimalarials, methotrexate).

APPENDIX 35

Electrocardiogram

Cardiac monitoring in suspected cases is an important part of physical health monitoring of mental patients. Every psychiatrist should take a correct decision about cardiac status by examining the ECG at outpatient department (OPD). Before prescribing a psychotropic drug, anti-ADHD drugs, one should carefully assess its risks and benefits to avoid any type of cardiac adverse reaction. The electroencephalogram (ECG) and electrolytes should be regularly monitored in patients taking psychotropic drugs.

On electroencephalogram (EEG) paper (marked with a grid of small and large squares). *Time* is measured along horizontal axis; each small square is 1 mm in length and represents 0.04 sec. Each larger square is 5 mm in length and represents 0.2 sec. *Voltage* is measured along the vertical axis; 10 mm is equal to 1 mV in voltage. The "height" of an ECG wave is called its **amplitude**. The isoelectric or baseline is a straight line and is considered to have an amplitude of zero. Anything above the isoelectric line is positive; below the line is negative.

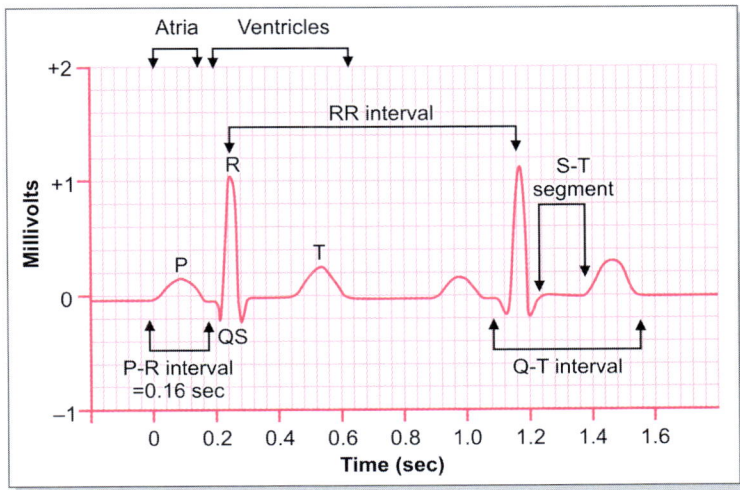

Source: HubPages. How to read a normal ECG electrocardiogram. [online]. Available from https://hubpages.com/health/How-to-read-a-normal-ECGElectrocardiogram [Accessed January 2019].

There are six limb [I, II, III, augmented Vector Right (aVR), augmented Vector Left (aVL), augmented Vector Foot (aVF) leads and six precordial (V1–V6) leads]. The usual paper speed is 25 mm/sec, i.e. there are 25 small squares in one second. The time interval measured by a horizontal 1 mm small square is thus 1/25 sec, i.e. 0.04 seconds (or 40 ms). If the paper speed is increased to 50 mm/sec, the horizontal distance of one small square measures 1/50 sec, i.e. 0.02 sec (20 ms).

The ECG records the fluctuations in electrical potential generated by the sequential *depolarization* and *repolarization* of the heart. There are three phases as follows:

1. *Atrial activation*: Depolarization *of the* atria generates a low amplitude wave; the **P wave**.
2. *Ventricular activation*: Once the excitatory impulse has depolarized then *ventricular* myocardium generate a complex waveform; the **QRS complex**. It is the largest ECG signal because of the larger muscle mass of ventricles.
3. *Recovery wave*: Ventricular *repolarization* then produces a prominent deflection in the ECG; the **T wave**.

■ NORMAL ECG WAVES, INTERVAL AND SEGMENTS (FIG. ABOVE)

P wave	• It is a small upward deflection representing atrial depolarization • It is upright in leads I, II, aVF, and V2–V6 and inverted in aVR • P wave is an upright, biphasic, flat, or inverted in V1, occasionally in lead V2
QRS complex	Q wave is a small downward deflection that follows P wave and represents depolarization of the interventricular septum • R wave is an upward deflection that follows Q wave • S wave is a small downward deflection that follows the R wave and represents ventricular depolarization • QRS is positive in all leads except aVR • Normal range up to 120 ms (3 small squares on ECG paper)
T wave	• It is an upward wave that follows the QRS complex • It represents ventricular repolarization. It is upright in all leads except aVR and V1
U wave	• It is a small wave that follows the T wave in the same direction • They represent repolarization of the papillary muscles or Purkinje fibers • It is best seen in lead V2 and V3
PR interval	• The time from the beginning of the P wave to the beginning of the QRS complex • Normal range 120–200 ms (3–5 small squares on ECG paper)
PR segment	• From the end of the P wave to the beginning of the QRS complex • It is isoelectric and acts as a baseline to evaluate depression or elevation of the ST segment. Normal range ~ 50–120 ms
QT interval	• Measured from the beginning of the QRS complex to the end of the T wave in leads II and V5–V6 • It indicates the time taken for ventricular depolarization and repolarization. Normal range up to 440 ms (though varies with heart rate and may be slightly longer in females)

Contd...

Contd...

QTc interval/Corrected QT interval	- It estimates the QT interval at a heart rate of 60 bpm - This correction allows comparing QT intervals over time at different heart rates and also improves detection of patients at risk of ventricular arrhythmia - The most frequently used formula to estimate QTc interval is Bazett's formula - *Bazett's formula* states QTc = QT/√RR where QTc = Corrected QT interval, QT = Uncorrected QT interval, and RR = RR interval - The normal QTc interval is 390–450 ms in men and 390–460 ms in women
ST segment	- It is the distance from the end of the S wave to the beginning of the T wave - It is usually isoelectric. Normal range: 80–120 ms
J point	- It is the point at which S wave joins the baseline - It is important in the evaluation of ST-segment deviation like ST elevation or depression
TP segment	- The portion between the end of T wave and the beginning of next P wave - At a normal heart rate, it is usually isoelectric and used as a baseline for determination of deviation of the ST segment
Ventricular activation time	- It is measured from the beginning of the Q wave to top of R wave - It should be <30 ms in leads V1–V2 and <50 ms in leads V5–V6

Features of Normal ECG

Rhythm	Sinus
Rate	60–100 beat per minute
Conduction	- PQ Interval: 120–200 ms/QRS width: 60–100 ms - QTc interval: 390–450 ms
Heart axis	Between -30 and +90 degrees
P wave morphology	- The maximal height of the P wave is 2.5 mm in leads II and/or III - The P wave is positive in II and AVF, and biphasic in V1 - The P wave duration is usually shorter than 0.12 sec
QRS morphology	- No pathological Q waves/No left or right ventricular - Hypertrophy/no micro voltage/normal R wave - Propagation (R waves increase in amplitude from V1–V5)
ST morphology	- No ST elevation or depression - T waves should be concordant with the QRS complex

QTc Interval

Long QT or QTc (calculated QT) intervals suggest abnormal effects on the myocardium. There are two types of QT prolongation:
1. *Congenital QT prolongation*: An inherited disorder which increases the risk of sudden cardiac death (SCD) of children or young adults

2. Acquired QT prolongation may be due to ischemia, electrolyte imbalance (hypokalemia or hypomagnesemia), CVA, medications of different types. Most acquired forms result from medications.
   Normal QTc Interval <440 ms
   Borderline QTc interval >440 ms but <500 ms
   Prolonged QTc Interval >500 ms

Extremely prolonged QT/QTcs can increase the patient's chances of SCD. The usual etiology of this death is Torsade de Pointes (TdP). When a patient has QT prolongation and bouts of syncope, TdP, or cardiac arrest, it is called "Long QT Syndrome" (Al-Khatib et al. 2003).

The potential for causing Prolonged QTc by psychotropic drugs (*Wenzel-Seifert et al. 2011*)

No effect on normal/ therapeutic doses	Mild effect (6–9 ms or only problems in overdose)	Moderate effect (10–15 ms)	Severe effect (>17 ms)
Antipsychotics			
Aripiprazole	Amisulpride	Risperidone	Quetiapine
Lurasidone	Flupentixol	Clozapine	Pimozide
Paliperidone	Olanzapine	Chlorpromazine	-
Zuclopenthixol	Haloperidol	-	-
Antidepressants			
Duloxetine	Citalopram/Escitalopram	Clomipramine	Amitriptyline
Mirtazapine	Trazodone	Fluoxetine	Doxepin
Sertraline	Venlafaxine		Imipramine
Fluvoxamine			Nortriptyline

Risk factors for QT prolongation and TdP (Wenzel-Seifert et al. 2011):
- Female sex (longer QTc interval than man and twice the risk of drug-induced TdP)
- Myocardial hypertrophy
- Congenital QT syndrome
- Bradycardia—2nd and 3rd-degree atrioventricular block
- Electrolyte disturbances (hypokalemia, hypomagnesemia)
- High plasma concentration of the offending drug because of overdose or intoxication.

APPENDIX 36

Some Clinical Syndromes

Amotivational syndrome—extreme lethargy, apathy, loss of interest and motivation, anergia and reduced drive, associated with chronic cannabis use.

Asperger's syndrome—a form of pervasive developmental disorder (usually associated with autism), characterized by significant difficulties in social interaction and nonverbal communication, along with restricted and repetitive patterns of behavior and interests and preoccupation with obscure facts.

Ganser's syndrome (hysterical pseudodementia)—approximate answer to questions though understands the nature of the question. Found in conversion disorder (hysteria), prison inmates.

Gilles de la Tourette's syndrome—onset in childhood, characterized by multiple motor tics and at least one vocal (phonic) tic. These tics characteristically wax and wane, can be suppressed temporarily, and are typically preceded by an unwanted urge or sensation in the affected muscles. Some common tics are eye blinking, coughing, throat clearing, sniffing, and facial movements.

Kleine-Levin syndrome (sleeping beauty syndrome)—a disorder characterized by persistent episodic hypersomnia and cognitive or mood changes. Many patients also experience hyperphagia, hypersexuality and other symptoms.

Neuroleptic malignant syndrome (NMS)—is a life-threatening idiosyncratic reaction to antipsychotic drugs characterized by fever, >38°C (>100.4°F), altered mental status, muscle rigidity, sweating and autonomic dysfunction. NMS is a ***medical emergency*** and can lead to death if untreated. Management includes stopping the offending medication, rapid cooling, and starting other medications. Medications used include dantrolene (post-synaptic muscle relaxant), bromocriptine (dopamine agonist) and diazepam. The syndrome is not dose-related and appears to be related to a very wide variety of substances including antidepressants, antipsychotics and lithium. There is a significant risk of mortality (about 10%).

Othello syndrome (conjugal paranoia)—where the content of delusions is predominantly jealousy (infidelity) involving spouse. This is a misnomer as Othello had no paranoid ideas but was deceived and acted on what was told to him regarding his wife (Crichton, 1996). The term should be abandoned.

Pickwickian syndrome (obesity- hypoventilation syndrome)—Sleep apnea more common in elderly and obese persons, associated with hypersomnia.

Locked-in syndrome—also called pseudocoma, where the patient is aware but cannot move or communicate verbally due to complete paralysis of almost all voluntary muscles except for vertical eye movement and blinking. It is caused by damage to areas in lower brain and brainstem with no damage to the upper brain.

■ SOME CULTURE-BOUND SYNDROMES IN INDIAN SUBCONTINENT

Dhat syndrome—patient complaints of a passage of 'dhat' (semen) in urine. Usually associated with multiple somatic symptoms, asthenia, anxiety, depression or sexual dysfunction (Prakash, 2007).

Gilhari (Lizard) syndrome—patient complaints of a subdermal swelling arising at the back, accompanied by apprehension and palpitation with shouting, crying and running spell with the fear of death as the swelling will reach the neck and causes difficulty in breathing. The cultural belief is that if the swelling which they believed as *Gilhari* is not crushed then they may die due to choked breathing. Crushed skin wound, made by faith-healer or relative of a patient is quite common (Jain et al. 2014).

Koro—affected male patient believes that his penis is shrinking and may disappear into his abdomen and he may die, associated with acute anxiety. An affected female believes that their breasts and vulva are shrinking. Occur in epidemic or sporadic form (Chowdhury, 1996).

Possession syndrome—patient is possessed usually by 'spirit/soul' of a deceased relative or a local deity. Patient speaks in a changed tone, even gender changes at times if the possessing soul is of opposite sex. Usually seen in rural areas. Majority of these patients are females who otherwise do not have any outlet to express their emotions (Chabra et al. 2008).

Appendix 37

Some Commonly Used Terms/Conditions in Clinical Psychiatry

Acculturation difficulty—a problem stemming from an inability to adapt to a different culture or environment appropriately. The problem is not based on any coexisting mental disorder.

Adherence/Compliance/Concordance—these terms are used in respect to medication taking behavior of a service user. WHO (2003) defines adherence as "the extent to which a person's behavior, taking medication, following a diet, and/or executing lifestyle changes, corresponds with agreed recommendations from a healthcare provider". In other words, it is the patient's agreement with the recommendations. Compliance implies patient passivity, which means acting in accordance with advice. Concordance is the fact of agreeing with the medical advice and reflecting the patient's responsibility. Though these words are used interchangeably in medication adherence assessment each of them has some different variables inherent in the concept (Aronson, 2007).

Advanced directives—are documents written while a person is competent specifying how decisions about treatment should be made if the person becomes incompetent.

Ambivalence—the coexistence of contradictory emotions, attitudes, ideas, or desires with respect to a particular person, object, or situation. Ordinarily, the ambivalence is not fully conscious and suggests psychopathology only when present in an extreme form.

Anaclitic—in psychoanalytic terminology, a dependence of the infant on the mother or mother substitute for a sense of well-being. This is considered normal behavior in childhood, but pathologic in later years.

Atypical or second-generation antipsychotics—include these chemical classes; dibenzoxazepine (e.g. clozapine), thienobenzodiazepine (e.g. olanzapine), and benzisoxazole (e.g. risperidone). These medications are known as "atypical" because they are generally more effective in symptom reduction than the earlier generation of antipsychotic medications, without the side-effect profile typical of those medications.

Avolition—an inability to initiate and persist in goal-directed activities. When severe enough to be considered pathological, avolition is pervasive and prevents the person from completing many different types of activities (e.g. work, intellectual pursuits, self-care).

Behavioral therapy—focusing on changing unwanted behaviors through rewards, reinforcements, and desensitization. Desensitization, or exposure therapy, is a process of confronting something that arouses anxiety, discomfort, or fear and overcoming the unwanted responses.

Catharsis—the healthful (therapeutic) release of ideas through "talking out" conscious material accompanied by an appropriate emotional reaction. Also, the release into awareness of repressed (forgotten) material from the unconscious, e.g. psychotherapy that encourages or permits the discharge of pent-up, socially unacceptable affects.

Caregiver—a person who has special training to help people with mental health problems, such as social workers, teachers, psychologists, psychiatrists, and mentors.

Case manager—an individual who organizes and coordinates services and supports for persons with mental health problems and their families.

Care plan—an agreement between the patient and the health professional (and/or social services) to help the patient to manage his/her health day-to-day. It can be a written document or something recorded in the patient notes. It will cover areas like the daily planning of activities, intended engagement with other support services, daily medicines, an eating plan, an exercise plan and emergency phone numbers to contact in a crisis.

Cognitive therapy—aims to identify and correct distorted thinking patterns that can lead to feelings and behaviors that may be troublesome, self-defeating or self-destructive. The goal is to replace such thinking with a more balanced view that, in turn, leads to more fulfilling and productive behavior.

Cognitive/behavioral therapy—a combination of cognitive and behavioral therapies that helps patients change negative thought patterns, beliefs and behaviors.

Comorbidity—the simultaneous appearance of two or more illnesses, such as the co-occurrence of schizophrenia and substance abuse or alcohol dependence and depression. The association may reflect a causal relationship between one disorder and another or an underlying vulnerability to both disorders. Also, the appearance of the illnesses may be unrelated to any common etiology or vulnerability.

Conventional or first-generation antipsychotics—a group of antipsychotic medications developed between the 1950's and 1970's; also referred to as "neuroleptics" or "traditional" or "classic" antipsychotics. These medications are effective for positive (psychotic) symptoms and less effective for negative symptoms and have varied side effects profile.

Covert medication—administration of any medical treatment in disguised form without the knowledge or consent of the person receiving it, for example in food or drink. It is done in a situation when the person lacks capacity regarding the medication taking, and covert medication is judged necessary after discussing it in the best interest meeting.

Cultural competence—is recognition of and response to cultural concerns of ethnic and racial groups, including their histories, traditions, beliefs, and value systems. It involves skills, attitudes and knowledge that allow persons, organizations and systems to work effectively with diverse racial, ethnic and social groups.

Disease-Course specifiers—single episode in full remission/single episode in partial remission/continuous/episodic with no inter-episodic residual symptoms/episodic with inter-episodic residual symptoms/unspecific.

Ego-dystonic—referring to aspects of a person's behavior, thoughts, and attitudes that are viewed by the self as repugnant or inconsistent with the total personality.

Ego-syntonic—denoting aspects of a person's thoughts, impulses, attitudes, and behavior that are felt to be acceptable and consistent with the self-conception. A good example is obsessive compulsive personality disorder which is ego-syntonic, as it is consistent with the way the patient thinks. On the other hand, obsessive compulsive disorder is considered to be an ego-dystonic disorder, as the thoughts and compulsions experienced or expressed are not consistent with the individual's self-perception, meaning the patient realizes the obsessions are not reasonable.

Evidence based medicine (EBM)—the "conscientious, explicit, judicious and reasonable use of modern, best evidence in making decisions about the care of individual patients. EBM integrates clinical experience and patient values with the best available research information" Masic et al. 2008. It is a sound clinical method that aims to increase the use of high-quality clinical research in clinical decision making. EBM requires new academic and clinical skills of the clinician, including efficient literature-searching and evaluation. The EBM practice is a process of lifelong, self-directed, problem-based learning by which the clinician is able to offer good quality clinical care to his/her patients with the updated expertise and knowledge about diagnosis, prognosis, therapy and other clinical and healthcare related issues.

First episode psychosis—refers to the first time that someone experiences psychotic symptoms or an episode. Schizophrenia and bipolar affective disorder usually appear when people are young (80% of first episodes of psychoses occur between 16 and 30 years of age), at a critical time in their intellectual and social development and thus requires early intervention (Shiers and Lesier, 2004).

Libido—is psychic drive or energy usually associated with the sexual instinct. "Sexual" is used here in the broad sense to include pleasure and love-object seeking.

Mood stabilizer—lithium and/or an anticonvulsant for treatment of bipolar disorder often combined with an antidepressant. Research has shown that treatment with an antidepressant alone increases the risk that the patient will switch to mania or hypomania, or develop rapid cycling.

Multidisciplinary—denotes an approach to care that involves more than one discipline. Typically, this will consist of doctors, nurses, social workers, psychologists and occupational therapists (multidisciplinary team).

Negative symptoms—most commonly refers to a group of symptoms characteristic of schizophrenia that includes loss of fluency and spontaneity of verbal expression, impaired ability to focus or sustain attention on a particular task, difficulty in initiating or following through on tasks, impaired ability to experience pleasure, to form emotional attachment to others, and blunted affect. The negative symptoms of schizophrenia can often appear several years before somebody experiences their first acute schizophrenic episode. These initial negative symptoms are often referred to as the prodromal period of schizophrenia.

Positive symptoms—commonly refers to a group of symptoms characteristic of schizophrenia that includes disorganized speech, confused thoughts (thought disorder), grossly disorganized or catatonic behavior, hallucinations and delusions.

Neurotic disorders—is mental disorder in which the predominant disturbance is a distressing symptom or group of symptoms that one considers unacceptable and alien to one's personality. There is no marked loss of reality testing, behavior does not actively violate gross social norms, although it may be quite disabling. The disturbance is relatively enduring or recurrent without treatment and is not limited to a mild transitory reaction to stress. There is no demonstrable organic etiology.

Object relations—emotional bonds between one person and another, as contrasted with interest in and love for the self; usually described in terms of capacity for loving and reacting appropriately to others. It is a theory of relationships between people, in particular within a family and especially between the mother and her child. A basic tenet is that we are driven to form relationships with others and that failure to form successful early relationships leads to later problems. It is also concerned with the relation between the subject and their internalized objects, as well as with external objects. Thus, we have a relationship with the internal mother as well as an external one.

Occupational therapy—uses goal-directed activities, appropriate to a person's age and social role, to restore, develop or maintain the ability for independent living (life skill development).

Placebo (or placebo effect)—is a fake treatment that does not contain any active substance to affect health, but a person has a response to that. This response may be positive or negative, called placebo effect. It depends on many factors like patient's expectations (positive thinking), his belief system and personality. To separate out this power of placebo effect of positive thinking from real benefit, the new drug trials have a placebo-controlled arm in its assessment of drug efficacy.

Psychotic disorders—are mental disorders in which the personality is seriously disorganized, and a person's contact with reality is impaired. During a psychotic episode, a person is confused about reality and often experiences delusions and/or hallucinations. Psychosis may be transient (hours or days) or persistent (months or years). The characteristic deficit in psychosis is not the "loss of touch with reality" but a loss of the ability to process experience appropriately that is an impairment of reality testing. The boundary between nonpsychotic and psychotic ideation and perception is not always sharp and clear. There is a spectrum from minimally distorted to grossly distorted nonpsychotic thinking, from mild impairment to severe impairment of reality testing, and from mild psychosis with circumscribed delusions to the extremely bizarre and disorganized psychotic state with complex delusions, hallucinations and behaviors.

Psychotherapy—a treatment method in which a mental health professional (psychiatrist, psychologist, counselor) and a patient discuss problems and feelings to find solutions. Psychotherapy can help individuals change their thought or behavior patterns or understand how past experiences affect current behaviors. There are several main broad systems of psychotherapy like psychoanalytic, psychodynamic, existential, humanistic, transpersonal, etc.

Primary gain—relief from emotional conflict and the freedom from anxiety achieved by a defense mechanism, e.g. alleviation of anxiety in neurosis by converting emotions into a somatic disease, a defense mechanism–hysterical dysphonia.

Prodrome—an early or premonitory sign or symptom of a disorder.

Reality testing—an ego function that enables one to differentiate between external reality and an inner imaginative world and to behave in a manner that exhibits an awareness of accepted norms and customs. Impairment of reality testing is indicative of a disturbance in ego functioning that may lead to psychosis. It is the most important ego function because it is necessary for negotiating with the outside world. Other functions are impulse control, affect regulation, judgement, object relations, thought process, defence reactions and synthesis.

Relapse—occurs when a person is affected again by a disease condition that affected him in the past.

Remission—is the state of absence of the disease activity in patients known to have the disease. It is commonly used to refer to the absence of active symptoms of the disease but may manifest again in the future. *Partial remission* is usually defined as 50% or greater reduction in the measurable parameters like symptom intensity, or biomarker levels (radiology, blood tests etc.). A *complete remission* is defined as complete disappearance of all manifestations of the disease.

Residual symptoms—some symptoms left behind, the disease has not been eradicated completely, also known as subsyndromal symptoms, e.g. between episodes, most people with bipolar disorder are free of symptoms, but as many as one-third have some residual symptoms. The presence of residual symptoms in remitted major depressive disorder patients has been associated with a greater risk of relapse, higher rates of suicidal attempts and ideation, and impaired functioning (Kennedy and Paykel, 2004).

Secondary gain—social, occupational, or interpersonal advantages that a patient derives from symptoms such as personal attention and service, monetary gains, disability benefits, and release from unpleasant responsibilities.

Sick role—identity adopted by an individual as a "patient" that specifies a set of expected behaviors, usually dependent. The concept of "sick role model" was designed by Talcott Parsons in the 1950s and was the first theoretical concept that explicitly concerned medical sociology. In contrast to the biomedical model, which regards illness as a mechanical malfunction or a microbiological invasion, Parsons described the sick role as a temporary, medically sanctioned form of deviant behavior.

Symptom—a subjective manifestation of a pathological condition. Symptoms are reported by the affected individual rather than observed by the examiner.

Signs—an objective indication of some medical fact or characteristic that may be detected by a physician during a clinical/physical examination of a patient. *Prognostic signs* indicate the outcome of the current bodily state of the patient. *Diagnostic signs* lead to the recognition and identification of a disease. *Pathognomonic signs* are the particular signs whose presence means, beyond any doubt, that a particular disease is present. *Premonitory signs* are the signs giving a warning for an incoming disease (aura before the seizure).

Syndrome—a grouping of signs and symptoms, based on their frequent co-occurrence, which may suggest common underlying pathogenesis, course, familial pattern, or treatment selection.

Treatment response—can be evaluated as a continuous measure, as a score on a rating scale (e.g. HAM-D), or as a category, such as improved, in remission, or relapsed. Response to treatment supposes that the therapeutic targets that have been defined a priori have been significantly modified by treatment. If rating scales are used, it is generally accepted that a change of less than 50% in the initial score is significant. Changes below that threshold will be considered as cases of nonresponse or insufficient response (Macher and Crocq, 2004).

[For Glossary of Mental Health Terms, useful in NHS/UK is available at www.malg.org.uk/documents/**glossary**.pdf]

Appendix 38

Mental Healthcare Act, 2017 (India)

On 28 March 2017, the Indian Parliament passed the Mental Healthcare Bill, 2016 which will be repealing the existing Mental Health Act, 1987. The bill was passed by the Rajya Sabha in August 2016. After receiving the assent of the President on the 7th April 2017, the Mental Healthcare Act, 2017 has come into existence. It has come in force with effect from 29th May 2018.

Mental Healthcare Act 2017—an Act to provide for mental health care and services for persons with mental illness (PMI) and to protect, promote and fulfill the rights of such persons during delivery of mental health care and services. It covers all disorders recognized by the WHO including alcohol and drug addiction, which the 1987 Act did not. Three landmark changes are Its clause on insurance; approach to treatment and decriminalization of attempted suicide. It has 16 Chapters and 126 Sections.

Chapter I:	Preliminary
Chapter II:	Mental Illness and Capacity to make Mental Healthcare and Treatment Decisions
Chapter III:	Advance Directive
Chapter IV:	Nominated Representative
Chapter V:	Rights of Persons with Mental Illness
Chapter VI:	Duties of Appropriate Government
Chapter VII:	Central Mental Health Authority
Chapter VIII:	State Mental Health Authority
Chapter IX:	Finance, Accounts and Audit
Chapter X:	Mental Health Establishments
Chapter XI:	Mental Health Review Boards
Chapter XII:	Admission, Treatment and Discharge
Chapter XIII:	Responsibilities of Other Agencies
Chapter XIV:	Restriction to Discharge Functions by Professionals not Covered by Profession
Chapter XV:	Offences and Penalties
Chapter XVI:	Miscellaneous

Some of the relevant provisions of the Act are:

Rights of a Person with Mental illness

Right to make an Advance Directive (Sections 5 to 13)—A person shall have the right to make an advance directive stating how to be treated and how not to be treated for the illness during a mental health situation.

Right to appoint a Nominated Representative (Sections 14 to 17)—A person shall have the right to appoint a nominated representative to take on his/her behalf, all health-related decisions.

Right to access mental health care (Section 18.1 and 2)—A person shall have the right to access to mental health care, treatment and services run or funded by the Government which are affordable, of good quality, in sufficient quantity, available nearby and without any discrimination.

Right to free services (Section 18.7)—A PMI living below the poverty line, a destitute or a homeless, shall get free treatment at state-run or funded health establishments.

Right to get quality services (Section 18.8)—The mental health services made available to PMI by the state shall be of the same quality as of general health services.

Right to get free medicines (Section 18.10)—All medicines on the essential drug list shall be made available to PMIs free of cost at the establishments run or funded by the government.

Right to community living (Section 19.1)—A PMI shall have the right to live in the community and be part of and not segregated from society.

Right to protection from cruel, inhuman and degrading treatment (Section 20.2)—Every PMI shall be protected from cruel, inhuman or degrading treatment in any mental health establishment (MHE).

Right to live in an environment, safe and hygienic, with basic amenities (Section 20.2.b, c and d)—Every PMI admitted shall have a right to safe and hygienic living environment, proper sanitation and facilities for leisure, recreation, education, religious practices and privacy.

Right to clothing (Section 20.2.e)—Every PMI living in an MHE shall have a right to proper and dignified clothing which prevents exposure.

Right to refuse work and get paid for the work done (Section 20.2.f)—No PMI shall be forced to work in an MHE, and those who agree to work shall be paid appropriate remuneration for the work done.

Right to protection (Section 20 k)—A PMI shall have protection from all forms of physical, verbal, emotional and sexual abuse.

Right to confidentiality (Section 23, 24)—All PMI has the right to confidentiality in respect of mental health, mental health care, treatment and physical healthcare. Photographs or any other information pertaining to the person cannot be released to the media without the consent of the person with mental illness.

Right to legal aid (27.1)—A PMI shall be entitled to receive free legal services to exercise his/her rights available under the Act.

Prohibited Procedures/Practices and Restrictions

No tonsuring (20.2.i)—No PMI in an MHE shall be subjected to compulsory tonsuring.

No compulsion to wear uniforms (Section 20.2.j)—A PMI shall not be forced to wear a uniform provided by the MHE.

No discrimination (21.1.a)—There shall be no discrimination on any basis including gender, sex, sexual orientation, religion, culture, caste, social or political beliefs, class or disability.

No electroconvulsive therapy (ECT) without anesthesia (Section 95.1.a)—ECT shall not be performed without the use of muscle relaxants and anesthesia.

Restriction on electroconvulsive therapy (ECT) for minors (Section 95.1.b and 95.2.)—ECT shall not be performed on minors. In exceptional cases, it may be done after getting informed consent of the guardian and prior permission of the Board.

No sterilization (Section 95.1.c)—Sterilization of men or women, intended as a treatment for mental illness, shall not be done.

No mechanical restrains (Section 95.1.d)—There shall be no chaining a person with mental illness, in any manner or form.

Restriction on psychosurgery (Section 96.1)—Psychosurgery shall not be performed as a treatment for mental illness without obtaining the informed consent of the patient and approval from the Board.

Restriction on physical restraints (Section 97.1)—Physical restraints shall be used sparingly, only when absolutely needed, and are deemed as the least restrictive method.

No solitary confinement (Section 97.1)—Seclusion and solitary confinement are totally banned.

Other Salient Provisions

Admission under this act may be made either as an "Independent" patient or as a "Supported Patient". The requirements for being admitted as a Supported Patient for up to one month and beyond one month are different. A minor can be admitted only on the application of his legal guardian or nominated representative. The admission and discharge procedures are discussed in Sections 86 to 90, the details of which should be consulted in the Act.

A small child to stay with inpatient mother (Section 21.2)—A woman receiving institutional care shall ordinarily not be separated from her child if the child is below the age of three.

Insurance cover for mental illness (Section 21.4)—Every insurer shall make provision for treatment of mental illness at par with provisions made for physical illness.

Emergency treatment (Section 94.1)—Any Registered Medical Practitioner can initiate emergency treatment to any person with mental illness if there is a threat to self, others, objects or property.

Protection to homeless persons with mental illness (section 100)—Officer in charge of a police station shall take under protection any person found wandering at large within the limits of the police station if he/she appears to be with mental illness and is incapable of taking care of himself/herself and will take him to the nearest mental health establishment within 24 hour for due assessment, treatment and subsequent action.

Police has also been given the responsibility (Section 101 and 102) to report about such mentally ill persons within his jurisdiction to the local magistrate, whom they think are either being ill-treated or neglected by their care-givers. The magistrate may order admission up to 10 days in a mental health establishment for assessment by the mental health professionals and subsequent course will follow after their assessment.

Attempt to commit suicide not an offence (Section 115.1)—A person who attempts to commit suicide will be presumed to be "suffering from severe stress" and shall not be subjected to any investigation or prosecution.

[Copy of the Act is available at http://www.prsindia.org/uploads/media/Mental%20Health/Mental%20Healthcare%20Act,%202017.pdf]

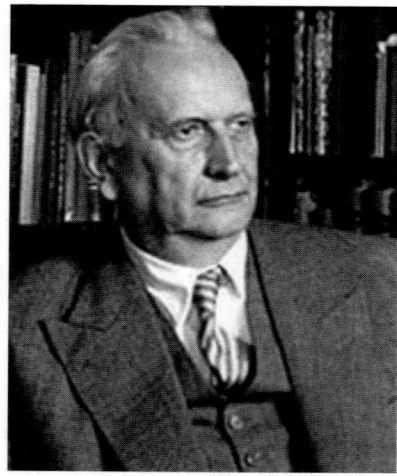

Karl Theodor Jaspers (23.02.1883–26.02.1969), a German psychiatrist and philosopher who immensely contributed to psychiatric phenomenology.

Bibliography

1. Ahmed SH. Cultural influences on delusion. Psychiatria Clinica. 1978;11:1-9.
2. Albrecht G, Sartore GM, Connor L, et al. Solastalgia: the distress caused by environmental change. Australasian Psychiatry. 2007;15(1):S95-8.
3. Al-Issa I. The illusion of reality or the reality of illusion: hallucinations and culture. Br J Psychiatry. 1995;166:368-73.
4. Al-Khatib AM, LaPointe NMA, Kramer JM, et al. What clinicians should know about the QT interval. JAMA. 2003;289(16):2120-7.
5. Amador XF, David AS. Insight, Culture and Society. In: Insight and Psychosis. London: Oxford University Press; 1998.
6. Amador XF, Gorman JM. Psychopathologic domains and insight in schizophrenia. Psychiatr Clin North Am. 1998;21:27-42.
7. American Psychiatric Association. Diagnostic and Statistical Manual for Mental Disorders, 4th edition. Washington DC: Text Revision, APPI.
8. Amnesty International UK. (2001) Universal Declaration of Human Rights. [online]. Available from https://www.amnesty.org.uk/universal-declaration-human-rights-UDHR [Accessed January 2019].
9. Anthony JC, LeResche L, Niaz U, et al. Limits of the 'Mini-Mental State' as a screening test for dementia and delirium among hospital patients. Psychol Med. 1982;12:397-408.
10. Arizmendi BJ, O'Connor MF. What is "normal" in grief? Aust Crit Care. 2015;28(2):58-62.
11. Aronson JK. Editors' view: Compliance, concordance, adherence. Br J Clin Pharmacol. 2007;63(4):383-4.
12. Beck AT. 1988. Beck Hopelessness Scale. The Psychological Corporation.
13. Berlin EA, Fowkes WC. Teaching framework for cross-cultural care: Application in Family Practice. West J Med. 1983;139:934-8.
14. Berrios GE, Porter R. A history of clinical psychiatry. In: The origin and history of psychiatric disorders. London: Athlone Press; 1995.
15. Binder RL. Are the mentally ill dangerous? J Am Acad Psychiatry Law. 1999;27:189-201.
16. Braham LG, Trower P, Birchwood M. Acting on command hallucinations and dangerous behavior: a critique of the major findings in the last decade. Clin Psychol Rev. 2004;24:513-28.
17. Brown S, Birtwistle J, Roe L. The unhealthy lifestyle of people with schizophrenia. Psychol Med. 1999;29:697-701.
18. Carlat DJ. The psychiatric interview. A practical guide. Philadelphia: Lippincott Williams & Wilkins; 1999.
19. Casey P, Kelly B. Fish's Clinical Psychopathology, 3rd edn. London: Royal College of Psychiatrists; 2007.
20. Cermolacce M, Sass L, Parnas J. What is bizarre in bizarre delusion? A critical review. Schizophr Bull. 2010;36:667-79.

21. Chabra V, Bhatia MS, Gupta R. Culture bound syndromes in India. Delhi Psych J. 2008;11(1):15-8.
22. Chapman LJ, Chapman JP, Rau-lin ML. Body-image aberration in schizophrenia. J Abnorm Psychol. 1978;87:399-407.
23. Chowdhury AN, Mukherjee H, Ghosh KK, et al. Puppy pregnancy in human: A culture-bound disorder in rural West Bengal, India. Int J Social Psych. 2003;49:35-42.
24. Chowdhury AN. Culture and posttraumatic stress disorder: a case of elephant attack. Dysphrenia. 2014;5(2):145-9.
25. Chowdhury AN. Culture, Psychiatry and Cultural Competence. In: (Ed: L L'Abate). Mental Illnesses - Understanding, Prediction and Control. London: InTech Publishers; 2011: pp. 69-104.
26. Chowdhury AN. Definition and classification of Koro. Culture, Medicine and Psychiatry. 1996;20:41-65.
27. Chowdhury AN. Koro. In: RL Cautin & SO Lilienfield (Eds). Encyclopedia of Clinical Psychology. 1st edition. New Jersey: John Wiley & Sons; 2015: pp. 1626-9.
28. Chowdhury AN. Mass hysteria with animal identification: Study from a tribal village in Tripura. J Indian Anthro Society. 1992;26:67-74.
29. Christodoulou GN. Syndrome of Subjective Doubles. Am J Psych. 1978;135:249.
30. Combs DR, Adams SD, Michael CO, et al. The conviction of delusional beliefs scale: Reliability and validity. Schizophr Res. 2006;86:80-8.
31. Cooper JE, Oates M. The principles of clinical assessment in general psychiatry. In: MG. Gelder, JJ. Lopez-Ibor, N.C Andreasen (Eds): New Oxford Textbook of Psychiatry. Oxford: Oxford University Press; 2000.
32. Cornell DG, Hawk GL. Clinical presentation of malingerers diagnosed by experienced forensic psychologists. Law Hum Behav. 1989;13:375-83.
33. Crichton P. Did Othello have 'the Othello Syndrome"? J Forensic Psych. 1996;7(1):161-9.
34. D Semple and R Smyth. Oxford Handbook of Psychiatry. UK: Oxford University Press; 2013.
35. Dening TR, Berrios GE. Autoscopic phenomena. British J Psych. 1994;165:808-17.
36. Denman C. Boundaries and boundary violations in psychotherapy. In: F Subotsky, S Bewley, M Crowe (Eds). Abuse of the Doctor-Patient Relationship. London: Royal College of Psychiatrists; 2010. pp. 91-103.
37. Department of Health. (2005). The Approach to be Taken in Response to the Judgement of the European Court of Human Rights in the 'Bournewood' Case. [online]. Available from https://webarchive.nationalarchives.gov.uk/+/www.dh.gov.uk/assetRoot/04/10/86/41/04108641.pdf [Accessed January 2019].
38. Department of Health. (2008). The Mental Capacity Act 2005, for use by the Oxford Radcliffe Hospitals NHS Trust', Susan Polywka, LSD- CGSU, February 2008, v2.i' www.southportandormskirk.nhs.uk/.../CLIN%20CORP%2061%20Mental%20Capacity%20Policy.
39. Diener E, Lucas RE. Personality traits. In: R Biswas-Diener and E. Diener (Eds). Noba textbook series: Psychology. Champaign, IL: DEF Publishers. 2018.
40. Dratcu L, Grandison A, McKay G, et al. Clozapine-resistant psychosis, smoking, and caffeine: managing the neglected effects of substances that our patients consume every day. Am J Therap. 2007;14:314-8.
41. DSM 5. Diagnostic and statistical manual of mental disorders. 5th Edition. Washington DC: American Psychiatric Association; 2013: pp.749-59.
42. Dubois B, Verin M, Teixeria-Ferreira C, et al. How to study frontal lobe functions in humans. In: AM Thierry, J Glowinski, PS Goldman-Rakic (Eds). Motor and cognitive functions of the prefrontal cortex. New York: Springer-Verlag; 1994: pp. 1-16.
43. Ellis HD, Whitley J, Luaute JP. Delusional misidentification:The three original papers on the Capgras, Frégoli and intermetamorphosis delusions. History of Psychiatry. 1994;5:117-46.

44. Epstein RS. Keeping Boundaries. Maintaining Safety and Integrity in the Psychotherapeutic process. Washington DC: American Psychiatric Press. 1994.
45. Eronen M, Hakola P, Tiihonen J. Mental disorders and homicidal behavior in Finland. Arch Gen Psychiatry. 1996;53:497-501.
46. Flaum M, Arndt S, Andreasen NC. The reliability of "bizarre" delusions. Comp Psychiatry. 1991;32:59-65.
47. Focus. Cultural Formulation: From the APA practice guideline for the psychiatric evaluation of adults, 2nd edition. Focus 2006. p.11.
48. Folstein MF. Mental state examination. J Psychiatric Res. 1975;12:189-98.
49. Freud S. Beyond the pleasure principle. Strachey J (Ed Trans). The standard edition. New York: WW Norton and Company; 1961.
50. Freudenreich O. Clozapine drug levels guide dosing. Curr Psychiatry. 2009;8:78.
51. Ganies AD. Culture-specific delusions. Sense and nonsense in cultural context. Psychiatric Clin North Am. 1995;18(2):281-301.
52. GMC. (2017). Confidentiality: good practice in handling patient information. [online]. Available from https://www.gmc-uk.org/guidance/ethical_guidance/confidentiality.asp [Accessed January 2019].
53. Goldberg D, Murray R. The Maudsley handbook of practical psychiatry. 5th edition. New Delhi: Oxford University Press; 2007.
54. Goldberg LR. An alternative description of personality: The Big Five personality traits. J Personality Social Psychology. 1990;59:1216-29.
55. Goldman RS, Emberger KM, Smet IC, et al. Cognitive neuroscience and neuropsychology. In: A Tasman, J Kay, JA Lieberman (Psychiatry Eds). West Sussex, England: Wiley & Sons Ltd.; 2004. pp. 363-402.
56. Goodwin DW, Anderson P, Rosenthal R. Clinical significance of hallucinations in psychiatric disorders: a study of 116 hallucinatory patients. Arch Gen Psychiatry. 1971;24:76-80.
57. Government of UK. (2005). Code of practice giving guidance for decisions made under the Mental Capacity Act 2005. [online]. Available from https://www.gov.uk/government/publications/mental-capacity-act-code-of-practice [Accessed January 2019].
58. Gutheil TG, Gabbard GO. The concept of boundaries in clinical practice: Theoretical and risk-management dimensions. Am J Psychiatry. 1993;150:188-96.
59. Guy W. Clinical Global Impressions (CGI) Scale, Modified. In: Task Force for Handbook of Psychiatric Measures. AJ Rush (Ed). 1st edition. Washington DC: American Psychiatric Association; 2000.
60. Hersh K, Borum R. Command hallucinations, compliance, and risk assessments. J Am Acad Psychiatry Law. 1998;26:353-9.
61. Hgiculescu RA. Therapeutic drug monitoring: which drugs, why, when and how to do it. Australian Prescriber. 2008;31:42-4.
62. Jacob R. Chowdhury AN. Assessment of mental capacity in patients recruited in clinical trials in psychiatry and its relationship to informed consent. Indian J Medical Ethics. 2009;6:43-4.
63. Jain A, Kumar KV, Omprakash J, et al. "Gilhari (Lizard) Syndrome" A New Culture Bound Syndrome. J Psychiatry. 2014;17:117.
64. Jaspers K. Zur Analyse der Trugwahrnehmungen (Liebhaftigkeit und Realittsurteli). Z Gesamte Neurol Psychiatr. 1911;6:450-535.
65. Junginger J. Command hallucinations and the prediction of dangerousness. Psychiatric Services. 1995;46:911-4.
66. Kasper BS, Kerling F, Graf W, et al. Ictal delusion of sexual transformation. Epilepsy and Behavior. 2009;16(2):356-9.
67. Kendler KS, Glazer WM, Morgenstern H. Dimensions of delusional experience. American J Psychiatry. 1983;140:466-9.

68. Kennedy N, Paykel ES. Residual symptoms at remission from depression: impact on long-term outcome. J Affective Disorder. 2004;80:135-44.
69. Kim SJ, Moon SW, Kim D. Body image distortions among inpatients with schizophrenia. Korean J Biological Psychiatry. 2012;19:211-8.
70. Kirmayer LJ. Cultural variations in the clinical presentation of depression and anxiety. Implications for diagnosis and treatment. J Clinical Psychiatry. 2001;62(13):22-8.
71. Klass ET. Situational approach to the assessment of guilt: development and validation of a self-report measure. J Psychopathological Behavior. 1987;9:35-48.
72. Kleinman A, Eisenberg L, Good B. Culture, Illness, and Care: Clinical lessons from anthropological and cross-cultural research. Annals Inter Med. 1978;88:251-8.
73. Kleinman A. Patients and Healers in the Context of Culture: An exploration of the borderland between Anthropology, Medicine and Psychiatry. Berkeley, California: University of California Press; 1981.
74. Kleinman A. Rethinking Psychiatry. New York: Free Press; 1988.
75. Kuruvilla K, Kuruvilla A. Diagnostic formulation. Indian J Psychiatry. 2010;52(1):78-82.
76. Lane C (2013). DSM 5 - Fifth Edition of The Diagnostic And Statistical Manual of Mental Disorders. Available at: http://www.psyweb.com/content/main-pages/dsm-5-fifth-edition-of-the-diagnostic-and-statistical-manual-of-mental-disorders
77. Laroi F, Luhrmann TM, Bell V, et al. Culture and hallucinations: Overview and future directions. Schizophrenia Bulletin. 2014;40(4):S213-20.
78. Laroi F, Somer IE, Blom JD, et al. The characteristic features of auditory verbal hallucinations in clinical and nonclinical groups: State of the art overview and future directions. Schizophrenia Bulletin. 2012;38(4):724-33.
79. Lee W, Cormac I. Meeting the physical health needs of people with mental disorders and disabilities. In: Essentials of physical health in psychiatry. I Cormac, D Gray (Eds). London: Royal College of Psychiatrists;. 2012; pp.3-13.
80. Leff J. The Unbalanced Mind. New York: Columbia University Press; 2001.
81. Leung WC, Passmore K. Essential notes for the MRCPsych Part 1. Berkshire, UK: Libra Pharm Ltd.; 2012.
82. Lewinsohn PM. An empirical test of several popular notions about hallucinations in schizophrenic patients. In: Origin and mechanisms of hallucinations (Ed W Keup). New York: Plenum Press; 1970. pp. 401-3.
83. Link B, Stueve A. Psychotic symptoms and the violent/illegal behavior of mental patients compared to community controls. In: Violence and Mental Disorder. J Monahan, HJ Steadman (Eds). Chicago, IL: University of Chicago Press; 1994: pp.137-59.
84. Lipsedge M. Clinical risk management in psychiatry. Quality in Health Care. 1995;4:122-8.
85. Mace C, Binyon S. Teaching psychodynamic formulation to psychiatric trainees. Part 1: Basics of formulation. Adv Psychiatric Treat. 2005;11(6):416-23.
86. Macher JP, Crocq MA. Treatment goals: response and nonresponse. Dial Clin Neur. 2004;6(1):83-91.
87. Malhi GS, Matharu MS, Hale AS. Neurology for psychiatrist. London: Martin Dunitz Ltd; 2000.
88. Mandelstan M. Safeguarding vulnerable adult and the law. London: Jessica Kingsley Publishers; 2009.
89. Masic I, Mikovic M, Muhamedagic B. Evidence based medicine—new approaches and challenges. Acta Informatica Medica. 2008;16(4):219-25.
90. McCall WV, Mann SC, Shelp FE, et al. Fatal pulmonary embolism in the catatonic syndrome: Two case reports and a literature review. J Clinical Psychiatry. 1995;56:21-5.
91. McKenna PJ. Disorders with overvalued ideas. British J Psychiatry. 1984;145:579-85.
92. Menzies RPD, Fedoroff JP, Green CM, et al. Prediction of dangerous behavior in male erotomanics. British J Psychiatry. 1995;166:529-36.
93. Mohl PC. Listening to patient. In: Psychiatry (Eds Tasman A, Kay J, Liberman JA). 2nd edition. Bangaluru: Panther Publication Pvt. Ltd.; 2004; pp. 3-18.

94. Mojtabai R, Nicholson RA. Interrater reliability of ratings of delusions and bizarre delusions. Am J Psychiatry. 1995;152:1804-6.
95. Mullen PE, Taylor PJ, Wessely S. Psychosis, violence and crime. In: Forensic Psychiatry: Clinical, Legal and Ethical Issues (Eds J. Gunn, P. Taylor). London: CRC Press; 1993; pp.329-71.
96. Mullen PE. Assessing risk of interpersonal violence in the mentally ill. Adv Psychiatric Treat. 1997;3:166-73.
97. Mulvey E. Assessing the evidence of a link between mental illness and violence. Hospital Community Psychiatry. 1994;45:663-8.
98. Mumenthaler M, Mattle H. Neurology. Germany: Georg Thieme Verlag; 2004; pp.2-5.
99. Nakaya M, Kusumoto K, Okada T, et al. Bizarre delusions and DSM-IV schizophrenia. Psychiatry Clin Neur. 2002;56:391-5.
100. Northfield J. (2004). Factsheet- what is learning disability. [online] Available from www.bild.org.uk/pdfs/05faqs/ld.pdf [Accessed January 2019].
101. Pandit MS, Pandit S. Medical negligence: Coverage of the profession, duties, ethics, case law, and enlightened defense—A legal perspective. Indian J Urology. 2009;25(3):372-8.
102. Perugi G, Ceraudo G, Vannucchi G. Attention deficit/hyperactivity disorder symptoms in Italian bipolar adult patients: A preliminary report. J Affective Disorder. 2013;149:430-4.
103. Pies RW. (2012). Bereavement and DSM-5, one last time. In Psychiatric Times. [online]. Available from http://www.psychiatrictimes.com/major-depressive-disorder/bereavement-and-dsm-5-one-last-time [Accessed January 2019].
104. Poole R, Higgo R. Psychiatric interviewing and assessment. New York: Cambridge University Press; 2006.
105. Prakash O. Lessons for postgraduate trainees about Dhat syndrome. Indian J Psychiatry. 2007;49(3):208-10.
106. Priebe S, Rohricht F. Specific body image pathology in acute schizophrenia. Psychiatry Research. 2001;101:289-301.
107. Rajagopal S. Catatonia. Adv Psychiatric Treat. 2007;13:51-9.
108. Rajender G, Kanwal K, Rathore DM, et al. Study of cenesthesias and body image aberration in schizophrenia. Indian J Psychiatry. 2009;51:195-8.
109. Richard M, Richard L. A comparison of delusions and overvalued ideas. J Nervous Mental Dis. 2010;198:35-8.
110. Rogers R. Assessment of malingering within a forensic context. In: Law and psychiatry: international perspectives. DW Weisstub (Ed). New York: Plenum Press; 1987; pp. 209-37.
111. Rohricht F, Priebe S. Do cenesthesias and body image aberration characterize a subgroup in schizophrenia? Acta Psychiatrica Scandinavica. 2002;105:276-82.
112. Roy RG. Cultural aspect of delusion. Arch Gen Psychiatry. 1962;7(3):219-20.
113. Royal College of Psychiatrists. (2007). Risk assessment and risk management in psychiatric practice. [online]. Available from http://www.rcpsych.ac.uk/pdf/Risk%20Assessment%20Paper%20-%20Giving%20up% 20the%20Culture%20of%20Blame.pdf [Accessed January 2019].
114. Royal College of Psychiatrists. (2009). Good psychiatric practice. [online]. Available from https://www.rcpsych.ac.uk/docs/default-source/improving-care/better-mh-policy/college-reports/college-report-cr154.pdf?sfvrsn=e196928b_2 [Accessed January 2019].
115. Royal College of Psychiatrists. (2016). Cultural psychiatry. [online]. Available from http://www.psychiatrycpd.co.uk/learningmodules/culturalpsychiatry.aspx [Accessed January 2019].
116. Rudnick A. Relation between command hallucinations and dangerous behavior. J Am Acad Psychiatry Law. 1999;27:253-7.
117. Severus WE, Kleindienst N, Seemüller F, et al. What is the optimal serum lithium level in the long-term treatment of bipolar disorder—a review? Bipolar Disorder. 2008;10:231-7.

118. Shapiro LJ, Stewart SE. Pathological guilt: A persistent yet overlooked treatment factor in obsessive-compulsive disorder. Annals Clin Psychiatry. 2011;23:63-70.
119. Shawyer F, Mackinnon A, Farhall J, et al. Acting on harmful command hallucinations in psychotic disorders: an integrative approach. J Ner Mental Dis. 2008;196:390-8.
120. Shiers D. Lester H. Early intervention for first episode psychosis. British Medical J. 2004;328:1451.
121. Silberman EK, Certa K. The psychiatric interview: settings and techniques. In: Psychiatry (Eds Tasman A, Kay J, Liberman JA). West Sussex: John Wiley & Sons Ltd.; 2004.
122. Simon M, Vörös V, Herold R, et al. Delusions of pregnancy with post-partum onset: an integrated individualized view. Euro J Psychiatry. 2009;23(4):234-42.
123. Singhal A, Kumar A, Belgamwar RB, et al. Assessment of mental capacity: who can do it? Psychiatric Bulletin. 2008;32:17-20.
124. Snyderman D, Rovner BW. Mental state examination in primary care: A review. Am Fam Physician. 2009;80(8):809-14.
125. Sommer IEC, Aleman A, Kahn RS. Left with the voices or hearing right? Lateralization of auditory verbal hallucinations in schizophrenia. J Psychiatry Neuro. 2003;28:17-8.
126. Swanson JW, Holzer C, Ganju VK, et al. Violence and psychiatric disorder in the community: evidence from the Epidemiologic Catchment Area surveys. Hos Comm Psychiatry. 1990;41:761-70.
127. Swanson JW, Swartz MS, Van Dorn RA, et al. A national study of violent behavior in persons with schizophrenia. Arch Gen Psychiatry. 2006;63:490-9.
128. Taylor D, Paton C, Kerwin R. The Maudsley Prescribing Guidelines. 9th edition. London: Informa Healthcare; 2007; p. 20
129. Taylor MA, Vaidya NA. Descriptive Psychopathology. New York: Cambridge University Press. 2009; p. 279.
130. Taylor PJ. Motives for offending among violent and psychotic men. British J Psychiatry. 1985;147:491-8.
131. Taylor PJ. When symptoms of psychosis drives serious violence. Soc Psychiatry Psychiatr Epidemiol. 1998;33(1):S47-54.
132. Teeple RC, Caplan JP, Stern TA. Visual hallucinations: differential diagnosis and treatment. J Clin Psychiatry. 2009;11(1):26-32.
133. The Journal of Family Practice. (2005). Feigned schizophrenia symptoms usually won't deceive the clinician who watches for clues and is skilled in recognizing the real thing. [online]. Available from http://www.jfponline.com/Pages.asp?AID=2821 [Accessed January 2019].
134. Thienhaus OJ, Piasecki M. Emergency psychiatry: Assessment of psychiatric patients' risk of violence toward others. Psychiatric Serv. 1998;49:1129-47.
135. Thompson JS, Stuart GL, Holden CE. Command hallucinations and legal insanity. Forensic Report. 1992;5:29-43.
136. Thorup A, Petersen L, Jeppesen P, et al. Frequency and predictive values of first rank symptoms at baseline among 362 young adult patients with first-episode schizophrenia: results from the Danish OPUS study. Schizophrenia Research. 2007;97:60-7.
137. United Nations Human Rights Office of the High Commissioner. (1965). International Convention on the Elimination of All Forms of Racial Discrimination. [online]. Available from https://www.ohchr.org/en/professionalinterest/pages/cerd.aspx [Accessed January 2019].
138. Urban M, Rabe-Jablonska J. Delusion of sex change and body dysmorphic disorder in clinical picture of paranoid schizophrenia—case reports. Psychiatria Polaska. 2010;44(5):723-33.
139. Urban-Kowalczyk M. Gender dysphoria as a clinical manifestation of schizophrenia- case series. Euro Psychiatry. 2015;30(1):1773.
140. Vaillant GE. Adaptation to life. Boston: Little, Brown; 1977.
141. Veale D. Over-valued ideas: a conceptual analysis. Behav Res Therap. 2002;40:383-400.

142. Velo GP, Minuz P. Medication error: prescribing faults and prescription errors. British J Clinical Pharmacol. 2009;67(6):624-8.
143. Voros V, Tenyi M, Trixler M. Clonal Pluralization of the self: A new form of delusional misidentification syndrome. Psychopathology. 2003;36:46-8.
144. Wahass S, Kent G. A cross-cultural study of the attitudes of mental health professionals towards auditory hallucinations. Int J Soc Psychiatry. 1997;43(3):184-92.
145. Wallace C, Mullen P, Burgess P, et al. Serious criminal offending and mental disorder: Case linkage study. British J Psychiatry. 1998;72:477-84.
146. Wechsler D. Wechsler Adult Intelligence Scale. New York: Psychological Corporation; 1955.
147. Weiss MG. Explanatory model interview catalogue (EMIC): Framework for comparative study of illness. Transcultural Psychiatry. 1997;34:235-63.
148. Wenzel-Seifert K, Wittmann M, Haen E. QTc prolongation by psychotropic drugs and the risk of Torsade de Pointes. Deutsches Arzeblatt International. 2011;108(41):687-03.
149. World Health Organization. (2017). ICD 11 Update. [online]. Available from http://www.who.int/classifications/ICD11January2017Newsletter.pdf?ua=1 [Accessed January 2019].
150. World Health Organization. Adherence to long term therapies: Evidence from action. (Ed Sabate E) WHO, Geneva, Switzerland. 2003.
151. World Health Organization. ICD-10 Classification of mental and behavioral disorders. New York: Churchill Livingstone; 1991.
152. Yager J, Gitlin MJ. Clinical manifestations of psychiatric disorders. In: Comprehensive Textbook of Psychiatry (Eds BJ Sadock, VA Sadock). 7th edition. Philadelphia: Lippincott Williams & Wilkins; 2000.
153. Zaman R, Makhdum A. Churchill's Pocketbook of Psychiatry. London: Churchill Livingstone; 2000; p. 41.
154. Zisook S, Shear K. Grief and bereavement: what psychiatrists need to know. World Psychiatry. 2009;8:67-74.

Photo of Lavater. Available at: http://en.wikipedia.org/wiki/Johann_Kaspar_Lavater
Photo of Esquirol. Available at : https://en.wikipedia.org/wiki/Jean-%C3%89 tienne_
Photo of Bonnet. Available at : http://en.wikipedia.org/wiki/Charles_Bonnet
Photo of GS Bose. Available at: https://en.wikipedia.org/wiki/Girindrasekhar_Bose

■ SUGGESTED READING

1. Bernstein CA, IsHak WW, Weiner ED, et al. On call psychiatry. 2nd Edition. WB Saunders Company: Philadelphia. 2001.
2. Bickerstaff ER. Neurological examination in clinical practice. 4th Edition. Blackwell Scientific Publications: London. 1980.
3. Goldberg D. The Maudsley handbook of practical psychiatry. Oxford University Press: New York. 1997.
4. Harrison P, Geddes J, Sharpe M. Lecture notes on Psychiatry. 8th Edition. Blackwell Science: Oxford. 1998.
5. Oyebode F. Sims' symptoms in the mind. An introduction to descriptive psychopathology. 4th Edition. Saunders Elsevier: London. 2008.
6. Strub RL, Black FW. The mental state examination in neurology. FA Davis Company: Philadelphia. 1995.

Index

A

Abnormal involuntary movement scale 171
Acathexis 90
Addiction severity index 171
Adult attention deficit hyperactivity disorder 132
    self-report scale 171
Aesop's fables 163
Affective disorders, schedule for 170
Aggression, episodes of 79
Agoraphobia 94
Agraphia 81
Alcohol 21
    abuse 58
    dependence, screening test for 171
    misuse of 55
    problems 59
    related problems 131
    withdrawal syndrome 108
Alcoholism 109
Alexia, pure 81
Alexithymia 90
Alkaline phosphatase 176
Alzheimer's disease 80, 89, 138
Ambitendency 7884
Amenorrhea 20
Amnesia 122
    anterograde 122
    dissociative 117123
    retrograde 122
    traumatic 122
Amnestic disorders 122
Amotivational syndrome 181
Amphetamine 21
Anankastic personality disorder 156

Anhedonia 89
Ankle 31
    clonus 31
Anorexia nervosa 97
Antipsychotics
    atypical 183
    conventional 184
    first-generation 184
    second-generation 183
Anton's syndrome 107
Anxiety 67
    disorder
        generalized 153
        separation 148
    episodic paroxysmal 153
    free floating 94
    general 170
    inventory 170
    neurotic 160
    reality 160
Anxious personality disorder 156
Aphasia 35, 80, 81
    anomic 80
    conduction 80
    expressive 80
    non-fluent 80
    phonemic 80
    pure 81
    receptive 80
    semantic 80
    type 81
Aphonia 82
Aprosodias 81
Aspartate aminotransferase 176

Asperger's syndrome 181
Ataxia, postural 33
Athetosis 30
Atonic seizures 77
Attention 46
   alternating 120
   and concentration 34, 46, 120
   deficit hyperactivity disorder 132, 171
   span 120
Attitude 5
   of parents toward sex 19
   toward opposite sex 19
Auditory verbal hallucination 112
Autism 89
   spectrum disorder 150
Autistic thinking 45
Autokinetic illusion 105
Autoscopy
   internal 109
   negative 109
Azotemia 85

B

Babinski response 32
Beck's depression inventory 136, 170
Beck's hopelessness scale 129
Beck's scale for suicide ideation 171
Beck's suicidal intention scale 129
Behavioral
   problems 18
   symptoms 67
   therapy 59, 184
Bender-Gestalt test 172
Bereavement exclusion, removal of 150
Biceps 31
Bilirubin 176
Binge eating 97
   disorder 149
Bipolar
   disorder 87, 88, 170
   graph 87
Birth
   complications 20
   history 17
   timing 20
Bizarre delusion 102
Blindness, cultural 72
Blood
   pressure 26
   urea nitrogen 176

Body
   dysmorphic disorder 96, 117 118
   image, distortion of 44, 117, 118
   mass index 74
      calculate 133
   system 16
Borderline personality disorder 88, 171
Brachial plexus 28
Bradylalia 83
Brain
   electrical activity in 115
   lesions 138
   neurochemical activity in 115
   tumors
      clinical features of 143
      general differential diagnosis of 143
Brainstem 142
   corticobulbar pathways in 142
Breathing 16
Brief psychiatric rating scale 137, 171
Broca's aphasia 80
Bulimia nervosa 97

C

Cage questionnaire 171
Calcium 176
Capgras delusion 100
Cardiovascular disease 74, 174
Cardiovascular system 26
Care plan 184
Catastrophic reaction 87
Catatonia 84
   malignant 85
Catatonic waxy flexibility 117
Catharsis 184
Central negative system, disorders of 114
Central nervous system examination 26, 27, 76
Central paresis 142
Cereal flexinilitas 84
Cerebellar disease 28, 33
Cerebral shock 28
Cerebrovascular disease 138
Cerebrum 142
Cervical
   cord tumor 28
   glandular enlargement 28
   rib 28
   spinal cord, upper 142
   spondylosis 28
   tumors 28

Charles Bonnet syndrome 111
Childhood disorders 18
Chloride 176
Cholesterol 176
Chorea 30
Clasp-knife spasticity 28
Clinical antipsychotic trials of intervention effectiveness 126
Clinical bedside frontal lobe tests 141
Clinical dementia rating 172
Clinical global impression-improvement scale 173
Clinical psychiatric evaluation and intervention, steps in 13
Clonus 29, 32
Clozapine 175
Clubbing 26
Cocaine 21
   intoxication 108
Cognitive
   development 19
   state assessment 138
   therapy 59, 184
Cogwheel rigidity 28
Coma 57, 76
   psychogenic 76
Communication
   attempt for 131
   nonverbal 5
   verbal 5
Complete blood count 174, 176
Composite international diagnostic interview 170
Comprehension, test for 36
Comprehensive psychopathological rating scale 171
Compulsion 94
Concentration, test for 46
Confusion 76
Conscious mind 158
Consciousness 27, 69
Convulsive movements 30
Cotard's syndrome 99
Couvade syndrome 102
Covert medication 185
Cranial nerves 27, 33
Crying, episodes of 79
Cryptamnesia 123
Cryptolalia 83
Cultural assessment, aim of 70

Culture-bound syndromes 182
Cyanosis 18, 26
Cyclothymia 89

D

Data Protection Act 12
De Clerembault's syndrome 99
Deafness, pure word 81
Decathexis 90
Deep tendon reflexes 32
Deep vein thrombosis 85
Delirium 76, 138
   common causes of 138
Delivery
   place of 18
   type of 18
Delusion 127
   amorous 99
   elicit nature of 41
   persecutory 98
Delusional misidentification syndrome 100
Delusional perception 110, 113
Delusional projection 161
Delusional thought 40, 98
   type of 40
Delusions
   different types of 98
   paranoid 98
Dementia 106, 123138, 172
   disability assessment for 172
   multi-infarct 138
Depression 67, 170
Depressive disorder 147
Dhat syndrome 182
Diabetes 26, 74
Disruptive mood dysregulation disorder 149
Dissociation 117162
Dissociative fugue 118123
Dissociative identity disorder 113, 118, 123
Distortion 161
Distress narratives 24
Domestic abuse 60
Domestic violence 60
Dominant parietal lobe tests 140
Dramatic cluster 155
Drugs
   attitude inventory 171
   misuse of 55

Dysarthria 35, 82
Dysgraphia 81
Dyskinesias 30
Dyslexia 125
Dyslipidemia, management of 75
Dysmegalopsia 104
Dysmorphophobia 96117
    delusions of 99
Dysphasia 82
Dysphonia 82
Dysphoric disorder, premenstrual 67
Dysprosody 35, 82
Dysthymia 89
Dystonia 30, 144
    levodopa-induced 30
Dystonic syndromes 144
Dystrophy, muscular 28

E

Eating disorders 59, 96, 133
Eccentric cluster 154
Echolalia 91117
Echopraxia 84117
Edema 26
Ego defense mechanisms 158, 161
Ego-dystonic 185
Ekbom's syndrome 99
Electrocardiogram 177
Electroencephalogram 144, 177
Electrolytes 176
Emotional abuse 60
Emotional problems, adolescent 19
Emotional status 171
Emotional symptoms 67
Emotionally unstable personality disorder 156
Emotions 114
Encephalopathy, metabolic 80
Epilepsy 30, 89, 138
    partial 30
Epileptic automatism 77
Erotic delusion 99
Excoriation disorder 149
Exhaustion 114
Extrapyramidal symptom rating scale 171
Extrapyramidal syndromes 143
Extraversion 69
Eye contact 78

F

Face and neck, involuntary movements of 30
Facial 27
    dystonia 31
    expressions 78
    tics 30
Fact feeling orientation 7
Fantasy 162
Fast speech 82
Federal Bureau of Investigation 98
Feeding habits 18
Financial abuse 60
Finger
    agnosia 140
    flexion 31, 32
    nose test 33
Fluent aphasia 80
Focal epilepsy 30
Folic acid 176
Folstein test 138
Forearm 28
Forensic problems 59
Forgetting 121
Formal thought disorder 39, 91
Foul body odors, delusion of 99
Free thyroxine index 176
Fregoli delusion 100
Frontal lobe
    functioning, assessment of 141
    syndrome 141
Frontal release signs 32
Functional level, assessment of 171
Fusion 91

G

Gait 29, 33
    ataxic 29
    high-stepping 29
    hysterical 30
    shuffling 29
    waddling 30
Ganser's syndrome 123, 181
Gastrointestinal system 26
Gender identity disorder 118
General health questionnaire 170
Genitourinary system 26
Genogram 66
Gilhari syndrome 182

Gilles de La Tourette's syndrome 181
Global aphasia 81
Glucose 174, 176
Grand mal epilepsy 30
Grandiose delusions 99
Grandiosity 95
Graphesthesia 31, 33
Grasp reflex 141
Growth and developmental targets 20
Guilt 93
    delusion of 57, 99

H

Halitosis 99
Hallucination 104, 115,115127
    auditory 107, 111, 113, 115, 116
    autoscopic 109
    causes of 114
    command 107, 112
    complex 106
        audiovisual 107
    elementary 106
    experiential 110
    extracampine 109
    fake 115
    frequency of 114
    functional 109
    gustatory 108
    haptic 108
    ictal 110
    imperative 107
    migrainous 109
    musical 109
    neurological causes of 145
    of bodily sensation 108
    olfactory 108
    organized 106
    panoramic 110
    proprioceptive 108, 109
    second person 111
    sexual 108
    tactile 108
    third person 111
    types of 107
    visual 107, 116
Hallucinosis
    organic 106
    peduncular 107
Halstead-Reitan battery 172

Hamilton rating scale 136
    for anxiety 170
    for depression 170
Harm, risk of 55
Head injury 80
Headaches 16
Hearing 16
Hebephrenia 151
Heel-knee test 33
Hematocrit 176
Hemiballismus 30
Hemiparesis
    clinical picture of 142
    lesions of 142
Hemoglobin 176
    glycosylated 176
Hepatitis B surface antigen 176
Hepatolenticular degeneration 144
Heroin 21
Hoarding disorder 149
Hoffman's reflex 32
Homicidal ideation 93
Hopelessness 93
Horn cell, anterior 28
Humor 163
Huntington's disease 89
Hypermnesia 122
Hypersomnia 65
Hypertension 16
    reduction of 75
Hypertonia, types 28
Hypervigilance 120
Hypnosis 114
Hypochondriacal delusion 100
Hypochondriasis 96162
Hypomania 153
Hyporeflexia 32
Hypotonia 28
    ipsilateral 28

I

Illness, explanatory model of 57, 71, 133
Infections 16
Infidelity, delusions of 98
Inflammatory lesions 28
Injury 16, 28
Insomnia 65
Institutional abuse 60
Intermetamorphosis 100

International Classification of Diseases 60, 151
International Classification of Epilepsy 77
Internet use gaming disorder 150
Interview
    clinical examination 1
    goal of 4
    management 1
    phases of 6
    process 5
    structure of 6
Interviewer
    attitude 5
    behavior of 5
Intravenous drug 21
Irritability 67
Isolation 163

J

Jargon aphasia 80
Jaundice 18, 26
Jaw jerk 31
Jealousy, delusions of 98
Joint pain 16

K

Kernig's sign 33
Kidney function test 176
Kleine-Levin syndrome 181
Knee 31
Korsakoff's syndrome 122

L

Labyrinthine disease 33
Lactate dehydrogenase 176
Language evaluation 34, 35, 80
Lead-pipe rigidity 28
Learning disability 59, 125
Lesion, site of 142
Lewy body disease 138
Libido 16, 185
Lipoprotein
    high-density 176
    low-density 176
    very low-density 176
Listening skill 5
Liver function test 174, 176
Lizard syndrome 182
Locked-in syndrome 57, 182

Logorrhoea 82
Lower limb 33
Luria-Nebraska neuropsychological battery 172
Lymphadenopathy 26

M

Magical thinking 92
Magnesium 176
Malignancy 28
Mannerisms 7884
Mass delusion 101
Masturbation, infantile 19
Material abuse 60
Mature defenses 163
Mean corpuscular
    hemoglobin 176
        concentration 176
    volume 176
Medical outcomes study short form 171
Memory 34, 47, 121
    autobiographical 121
    declarative 121
    disorders of 122, 124
    disturbances, psychogenic 123
    explicit 121
    functions of 121
    implicit 121
    long-term 121
    photographic 105
    procedural 121
    recent 48
    remote 48
    short-term 121
    topographic 121
    type of 121, 124
Menarche age 20
Meningeal signs 33
Menopause 20
Menstrual history 20
Mental capacity assessment 56
Mental disorder
    code, diagnostic and statistical manual of 60
    primary care of 170
Mental health
    establishment 190
    physical health monitoring in 74
Mental Healthcare Act 2017 189
Mental illness, rights of person with 190
Mental State Examination 26, 34, 57, 72

Metabolic syndrome 74
   management of 75
Metonyms 91
Millon clinical multiaxial inventory 171
Mini-cog test 140
Mini-Mental State Examination 138
Minnesota multiphasic personality inventory 171
Montogomery-Asberg depression rating scale 170
Mood 38
   and affect 34, 38, 86
   congruent 110
   disorder
      family history of 58
      graph 88
      questionnaire 170
   incongruent 110
   stabilizer 185
   swings 67, 88, 89
      differential diagnosis of 88
      menopausal 89
   type 38, 86, 87
Moral
   anxiety 160
   behavior 34, 37
   development 19
   neurone disease 28
   perseveration 85
   sensory link 31, 33
   system 33
Muller-Lyer illusions 105
Multidisciplinary team 72
   and cultural formulation 72
Munchausen syndrome 96
Muscle
   power 29, 33
   tone 28, 33
   wasting 28, 33
      peripheral 28
      proximal 28
Mutism 83
Myoclonic jerks 30
Myoclonus 144
Myositis 28

N

National Institute of Mental Health 126
Neck rigidity 33
Nephropathy, obstructive 85
Nerve injury, peripheral 28
Neuroleptic malignant syndrome 181
Neuropsychiatric inventory 172
Neuropsychiatry 170
Neuropsychologic tests 172
Neurotic disorders 186
Neuroticism 69
Non-bizarre delusion 102
Non-suicidal self-injury 150

O

Obesity 26, 74
   hypoventilation syndrome 182
Obsessive
   compulsive disorder 109, 153
   personality traits 58
Occupational therapy 186
Oculomotor 27
Opisthotonus 30
Opium 21
Optic 27
Optical illusion 105
Oral glucose tolerance test 176
Organic brain disease 138
Organizational abuse 60
Othello syndrome 181

P

Pain 33
Palilalia 91
Pallor 26
Panic
   attacks, post-traumatic stress disorder 46
   disorder 153, 170
   inventory, acute 170
Paracusia 107
Paragrammatism 91
Paramnesia 122
   reduplicative 100, 122
Paranoia 95
   conjugal 181
   litigious 98
Paranoid personality disorder 156
Paraphasia 35, 83
Parasitosis delusion of 108
Parasomnia 65
Pareidolias 105

Paresis 142
   different types of 142
   peripheral 142
Parietal lobe
   disorders 140
   tests 140
Parkinson's disease 30, 89
Parosmia 108
Past-pointing test 33
Patellar clonus 31
Pedophilic disorder 150
Perioral tremor 30
Peripheral smear 176
Peroneal muscular atrophy 28
Persistent complex bereavement disorder 147
   differential diagnosis of 147
Personality
   disorder 59, 154, 156, 171
      histrionic 156
      ICD-10 classification of 156
      multiple 123
      specific 156
   premorbid 22, 60, 68
   status 171
   traits 68
Petit mal epilepsy 30
Phantageusia 108
Phantom limb 105
Phantosmia 108
Phobia 170
   simple 94
   social 94, 170
Phobic anxiety disorder 153
Phoneme 112
Phosphorus 176
Physical abuse 19, 60
Physical problems, adolescent 19
Pickwickian syndrome 182
Pierce suicide intent scale 171
Platelet count 176
Poliomyelitis 28
Polyneuritis 28
Positive and negative symptom scale 171
Possession syndrome 182
Post-traumatic stress disorder 105, 132, 147, 150
   clinician-administered 170
Potassium 176
Poverty, delusion of 99
Preconscious mind 158

Pregnancy 89
   delusion of 101
   false 101
   phantom 101
Premenstrual syndrome 67
   symptoms of 89
Primitive reflexes 32
Prothrombin time 176
Pseudocyesis 101
Pseudodementia, hysterical 181
Pseudohallucinations 110
Pseudologia fantastica 123
Psychiatric history 13, 14, 60
Psychiatric interview 3
   general features of 5
Psychiatric nurse 73
Psychiatric report 168
Psychiatric screening tests 170
Psychiatry
   commonly used
      laboratory tests in 174
      rating scales in 170
   cultural assessment in 70
   psychoanalytical 165
Psychological abuse 60
Psychological screening inventory 170
Psychomotor activity, level of 37
Psychosis 126, 171
   first episode 185
Psychotherapy 59, 187
Psychotic
   disorders 186
   state, acute 46
   symptoms 55
Psychotomimetic drugs 114
Pubertal development 20
Puberty
   onset of 19
   through adolescence 18
Pulse 26
Pyramidal tract lesion 33

Q

Querulous 98

R

Random plasma glucose 176
Rape, delusion of 102
Rating scale 136

Raven's progressive matrices 172
Reaction formation 163
Reality testing 187
Red blood cell count 176
Reflex 31, 33
　arc 28
　hallucinations 109
　superficial 32
Regression 163
Respiratory system 26
Retention loss 121
Retrospective falsification 123
Royal College of Psychiatrist 75

S

Scale for assessment of
　negative symptoms 171
　positive symptoms 171
Schizoid personality disorder 156
Schizophrenia 34, 85, 109, 111, 137, 150, 151, 170, 171
　catatonic 85
　section of 151
　symptoms in 113, 146
　type of 151
School life and academic achievements 20
Sclerosis, multiple 89
Seductive behavior 131
Seizures
　absence 77
　complex partial 77
　episode, different stages of 77
　generalized 77
　myoclonic 77
　partial 77
　simple partial 77
　unclassified 77
Self-harm
　inventory 171
　thought 93
Sensations, proprioceptive 31
Sensory
　ataxia 33
　deprivation 114
　inattention 33
　　test for 31
　system 31, 33
Serotonin syndrome 32, 77
Serum gamma-glutamyl transferase 176
Serum glutamic-pyruvic transaminase 176

Serum lithium estimation 175
Sex change, delusion of 102
Sexual abuse 19, 60
Sexual activity, adolescent 19
Sexual exploitation 60
Sexual knowledge, acquisition of 19
Sexual practices 19
Sexual symptoms 19
Sexual therapy 59
Sexuality, adult 19
Sick role 188
Side effects scale 171
Simpson-Angus scale 171
Sin 93
Six-item cognitive impairment test 140
Skin 16, 26
Sleep 16
　deprivation 114
　disorders 65
　rhythm problem 65
Sleeping beauty syndrome 181
Social anxiety 170
Social readjustment rating scale 171
Sodium 176
Solastalgia 90
Somatic delusions 99
Somatization 162
Spasmodic torticollis 31, 144
Specific learning disorder 150
Speech 27, 34, 36, 82
　abnormalities 85
　nonspontaneous 82
　poverty of 82, 91
　　content of 82
　pressure of 82
　push of 82
　slow 82
　slurring 83
　telegraphic 83
Spinal accessory 27
Spinal cord, corticospinal pathways in 142
Spinal shock 28
Spine 26
State-trait anxiety inventory 170
Stereognosis 31, 33
Stereotypy 84, 91
Stress 114
　significant 55
Stupor 7684
Substance use disorder 59, 150

Suicidal ideation ever, acute 21
Suicidal intent 129
Suicidal thought 93
Suicide 54
    attempts, inventory of motivations for 129
    risk 136
        assessment 136
Superior pulmonary sulcus tumor 28
Supinator 31
Suppression 164
Surrogate consent 12
Synesthesia 109
Syphilis 138
Syringomyelia 28
Systemic examination 26

T

Tardive dyskinesia 145
Taste 16
Tension, intracranial 143
Therapeutic drug monitoring 174
Therapeutic medication, rearrangement of 75
Therianthropy 103
Thinking, abstract 34, 44
Third person auditory hallucination 57
Thought 93
    alienation 92
    broadcasting of 92, 113
    control 92
    diffusion 92
    echo 92
    insertion 92
    interference, delusions of 113
    non-delusional 93
    racing 91
    system, examination of 39
    withdrawal 92
Thyroid 26
    function test 176
    problems 16
    stimulating hormone 176
Thyrotoxicosis 28
Thyroxine 176
Tobacco 21
    smoking 26
Tonic-clonic seizures 77
Torsion dystonia 144

Transient global amnesia 122
Tremors 26
Triglycerides 176
Tri-iodothyronine 176
Trouble with urination 16

U

Upper limb 33
Uric acid 176
Urine analysis 176

V

Vagus 27
Vascular accident 28
Vegetative signs 65
Ventricular activation 178
Verbal fluency 36
    test for 36
Vigilance 120
Violence, risk 55
    factors for 126
Vision 16
Visual analog scale 172
Visual hallucination
    clinical picture of 107
    features of 107
Voice 34, 36, 82, 112
    content of 112

W

Wasting, generalized 28
Waxy flexibility 84
Wechsler adult intelligence scale 172
Weight gain, drugs associated with 74
Wender Utah rating scale 171
Wernicke's aphasia 80
Wernicke's encephalopathy 122, 138
Wernicke-Korsakoff syndrome 122, 123
White blood cell count 176
Wilson's disease 144
World Health Organization 125
    Quality of Life 171

Y

Yale-brown obsessive-compulsive scale 170
Young mania rating scale 170